W0227878

Manual of Tropical Dermatology

John H. S. Pettit
Lawrence Charles Parish

Manual of
Tropical Dermatology

With 119 Figures and 12 Color Plates

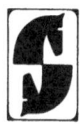

Springer-Verlag
New York Berlin Heidelberg Tokyo

John H.S. Pettit, M.D., F.R.C.P. (London), Department of Tropical Medicine, Liverpool School of Tropical Medicine, Liverpool, England; and Department of Medicine, Universiti Kebangsaan, Kuala Lumpur, Malaysia.

Lawrence Charles Parish, M.D., F.A.C.P., Department of Dermatology, Jefferson University, Philadelphia, Pennsylvania 19107; and Division of Dermatology, University of Pennsylvania, School of Veterinary Medicine, Philadelphia, Pennsylvania, 19104, U.S.A.

Library of Congress Cataloging in Publication Data
Pettit, John H. S.
    Manual of tropical dermatology.
    Bibliography: p.
    Includes index.
    1. Dermatology—Handbooks, manuals, etc. 2. Tropical
medicine—Handbooks, manuals, etc. I. Parish, Lawrence
Charles. II. Title.
RL74.P48 1984   616.5′00913   94-5323

© 1984 by Springer-Verlag New York, Inc.
Softcover reprint of the hardcover 1st edition 1984

All rights reserved. No part of this book may be translated or reproduced in any form without written permission from Springer-Verlag, 175 Fifth Avenue, New York, New York 10010, U.S.A.
The use of general descriptive names, trade names, trademarks, etc., in this publication, even if the former are not especially identified, is not to be taken as a sign that such names, as understood by the Trade Marks and Merchandise Marks Act, may accordingly be used freely by anyone.

While the advice and information of this book is believed to be true and accurate at the date of going to press, neither the authors nor the editors nor the publisher can accept any legal responsibility for any errors or omissions that may be made. The publisher makes no warranty, express or implied, with respect to material contained herein.

Typeset by University Graphics, Incorporated, Atlantic Highlands, New Jersey.

9 8 7 6 5 4 3 2 1
ISBN-13:978-1-4613-8294-2   e-ISBN-13: 978-1-4613-8292-8
DOI: 10.1007/978-1-4613-8292-8

Dedicated to two of our favorite teachers and colleagues:

Geoffrey B. Dowling, M.D., F.R.C.P., (London) (deceased), Dermatologist, St. Thomas Hospital, London, and St. John's Hospital Diseases of the Skin, London
and
Herman Beerman, M.D., Sc.D., F.A.C.P., Emeritus Professor of Dermatology, University of Pennsylvania School of Medicine and Emeritus Professor and Chairman, Department of Dermatology, University of Pennsylvania Graduate School of Medicine, Philadelphia, Pennsylvania.

Contents

Foreword
Francisco Kerdel-Vegas   ix
Preface   xi
Acknowledgments   xiii

I   Introduction

   1   Introduction to Tropical Dermatology   3
   2   Clinical Index   6

II Bacterial Diseases

   3   Anthrax   21
   4   Yaws   27
   5   Tuberculosis of the Skin   36
   6   Leprosy   47
   7   Buruli Ulcer (Mycobacterium Ulcerans)   78
   8   Tropical Ulcers   88

III Fungal Diseases

   9   Tropical Tineas   95
  10   Chromomycosis   106
  11   Madura Foot and Other Mycetomas   112
  12   Sporotrichosis   118
  13   Actinomycosis   124
  14   Botryomycosis   129
  15   Rhinosporidiosis   133
  16   Rhinoscleroma   137
  17   North American Blastomycosis   141
  18   Paracoccidioidomycosis   146
  19   Lobo's Disease   152

IV   Parasitic Diseases

20   Leishmaniasis   159
21   Amebiasis   178
22   Toxoplasmosis   183
23   Onchocerciasis   187
24   Filariasis   195
25   Dracunculosis   200
26   Schistosomiasis   205

V   Other Dermatoses

27   Lichen Planus Tropicus   215
28   Dietary Deficiencies   221
29   Phrynoderma   228
30   Brazilian Pemphigus Foliaceous   232
31   Chronic Arsenical Poisoning   238

Appendix One   Useful Techniques   243

Appendix Two   Useful Addresses   250

Index   253

Foreword

We live today in a world densely populated by human beings living in close communication with one another all over the surface of the planet. Viewed from a certain distance it has the look of a single society, a community, the swarming of an intensely social species trying to figure out ways to become successfully independent. We obviously need, at this stage, to begin the construction of some sort of world civilization. The final worst-case for all of us has now become the destruction, by ourselves, of our species.[1]

Although this warning is often repeated, we must not forget its paramount importance and the commitment that each sector of society has to make a *world civilization* possible.

Tropical dermatology is a good example of an important area of our specialty that has never caught the proper attention of the leading centers of research in the developed countries, even though it comprehends major infectious, parasitic, and nutritional problems of one-half of the world's land area and three-quarters of the world's population.

The relevance of tropical dermatology in this extensive and overpopulated area of the globe has public health connotations that emphasize its importance. The sheer size of the problem makes it an urgent and outright need to recruit and train adequate personnel to do a proper job, and that includes not only dermatologists but paramedical personnel, nurses, and laboratory technicians.

This book written by John H. S. Pettit and Lawrence Charles Parish is precisely the type of guidance needed by the uninitiated, presented in a logical and intelligent manner so it can be used throughout the world as a training manual. Such initiative is welcome and needed, and complements very well other efforts in the same direction.

Even in tropical countries, tropical dermatology does not occur everywhere, and the ordinary tourist, staying in a metropolitan hotel, rarely becomes exposed to what were once called exotic diseases. The moment the pleasures of

---

[1]Lewis Thomas: *Late Night Thoughts on Listening to Mahler's Ninth Symphony*. New York, Viking Press, 1983.

a big city are left behind, however, it seems that, in the rural areas of many developing countries and in this century of unprecedented scientific and technologic advances, most people remain living under conditions that have not changed for centuries and suffering from a host of infecious and contagious diseases that are the main obstacle to any program designed to improve their lives.

It is the duty of the medical profession, and in this case the dermatologists, to study these problem with the greatest attention and coherence and to produce a strategy to overcome this burden in a short period of time. What has been done until now is not sufficient and the problem remains unsolved.

Francisco Kerdel-Vegas, M.D.
Caracas, Venezuela and
Department of Dermatology
Jefferson Medical College
Thomas Jefferson University
Philadelphia, Pennsylvania
U.S.A.

Preface

When the world was young and transport was difficult, most people lived their lifetime without venturing far from home. Migrants were few, whether they traveled on foot, on horseback, or by boat, but those who did travel carried their diseases with them as well as other more accepable examples of their culture. The unacceptable ones often led to war, an additional method of spreading disease.

As travel has become easier, diseases have become increasingly widespread, but unfortunately knowledge of such illnesses has not extended as rapidly as the diseases themselves. This book has been so conceived that it will aid in the recognition and treatment of some of the more exotic of the world's diseases.

September, 1984

John H. S. Pettit, M.D.
Lawrence Charles Parish, M.D.

Acknowledgments

We want to acknowledge the magnificent resource material available at the Library of the College of Physicians of Philadelphia (Anthony Aguirre, librarian) and the Scott Medical Library of the Jefferson Medical College, Thomas Jefferson University (John Timour, librarian).

Although many of the illustrations are of our own patients, we have called upon a number of colleagues throughout the world for their assistance. Our most heartfelt thanks to all of them; all such collaborators are acknowledged under the appropriate pictures. We hope we have not missed any.

Dr. Florante C. Bocobo, Princeton, New Jersey reviewed the chapters on actinomycosis and North American blastomycosis. Dr. Joseph Scrafani, Schering-Plough Corporation, Kenilworth, New Jersey provided a grant-in-aid for the production of the color plates.

Lastly, we wish to thank Carmela Ciferni and Margaret DiFrancesco of Philadlephia for working through this project and typing the manuscript.

Color Plates

Plate 1   Ulcer, lepromatous—Note the granulation tissue in the ulcer on the sole and the lack of surrounding erythema. This Malaysian patient had lepromatous leprosy.

Plate 2   Ulcer, phagedenic—Note the extending margins of this patient with a phagedenic ulcer of the foot. The diagnosis was tropical ulcer.

Plate 3   Verrucous formation—Note the warty heaped-up lesions, reddish, and slightly scaling on the buttocks of a Chinese man. The diagnosis was tuberculosis verrucosa cutis.

Plate 4   Sun sensitivity—Note the symmetrical reddish-brown pigmentation with sharp borders indicating the photosensitive areas. This Egyptian woman had pellagra. (Courtesy of Mohsen Soliman, M.D., Cairo, Egypt.)

Plate 5   Erosion, ear—Note the destruction, ulceration, and surrounding erythema on the upper aspects of the outer ear. This Philadelphia anthropology student had contracted chiclero ulcer on a dig.

Plate 6   Papules, coalescent—Note the coalescent papules with purplish color. This Italian man was sun sensitive and developed lichen planus tropicus. (Courtesy of F. Ayala, M.D., Naples, Italy.)

Plate 7   Ulcer, Buruli—Note the destruction with shaggy borders on the ankle. This Malaysian aborigine first developed swelling seven months before the ulcer appeared.

Plate 8   Nodules, heaped-up—Note the heaped-up, shiny lesions in this patient with lepromatous leprosy which was sulfone resistant.

Plate 9   Ulcer, penile—Note the granulomatous formation at the edge of the ulcer, which is somewhat shaggy. This North Carolina man had North Americn blastomycosis. (Courtesy of David M. Warshauer, M.D., Chapel Hill, North Carolina.)

Plate 10   Verrucous formation—Note the warty papules that have coalesced and have become covered with thick scale and the sharp borders of the lesions on the foot of this 58 year old Indian man who worked barefoot on a farm. The diagnosis was chromomycosis.

Plate 11   Keratoses—Note the crusting, scaling, and hyperkeratoses characteristic of arsencial keratoses. This Malay youth had used a Thai folk remedy containing 21.5% arsenic.

Plate 12   Scarring—Note the destructive atrophic scars in this Iranian patient with lupoid leishmaniasis.

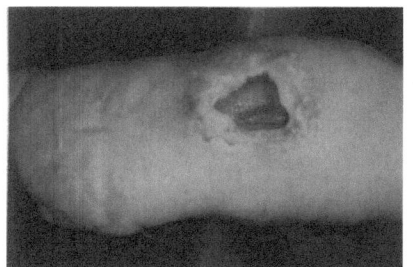

Plate 1 Ulcer, lepromatous

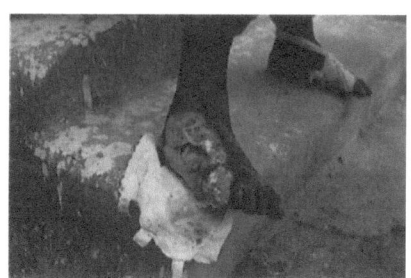

Plate 2 Ulcer, phagedenic

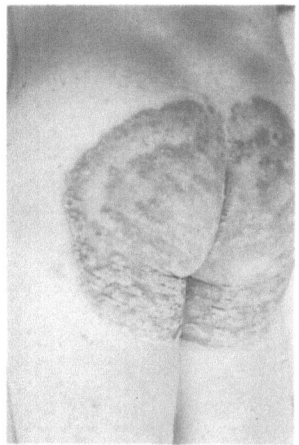

Plate 3 Verrucous formation

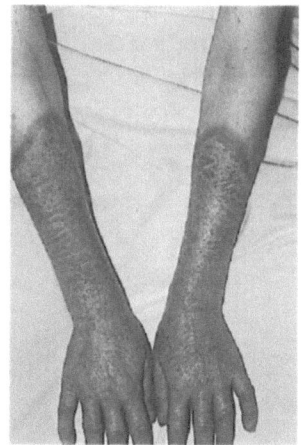

Plate 4 Sun sensitivity

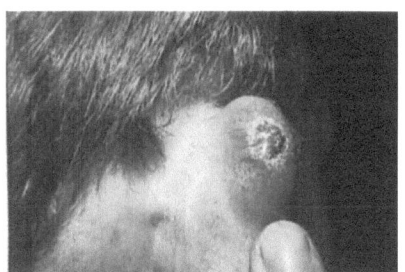

Plate 5 Erosion, ear

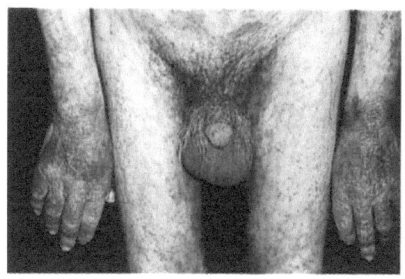

Plate 6 Papules, coalescent

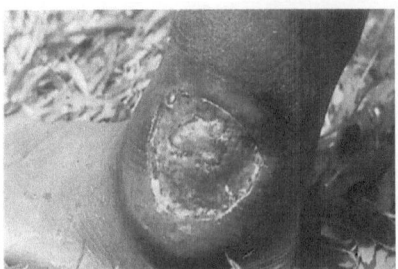

Plate 7   Ulcer, Buruli

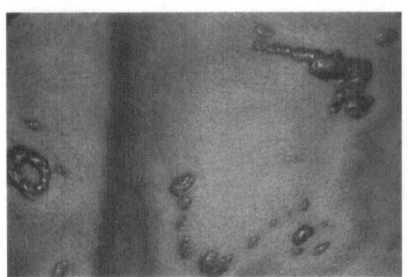

Plate 8   Nodules, heaped-up

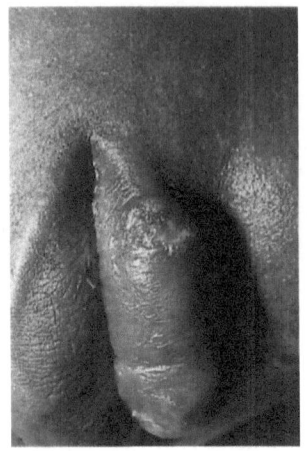

Plate 9   Ulcer, penile

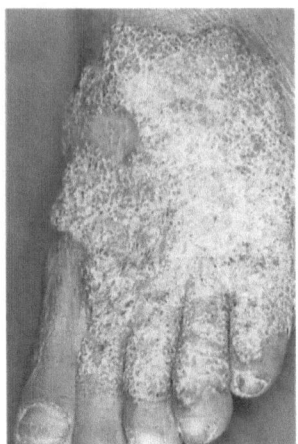

Plate 10   Verrucous formation

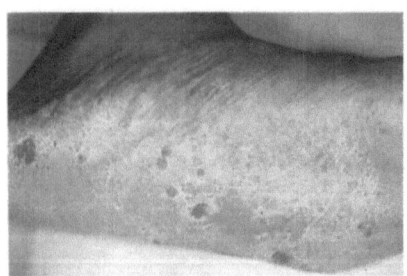

Plate 11   Keratoses

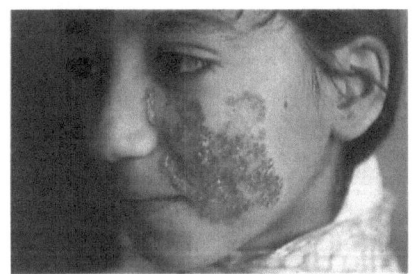

Plate 12   Scarring

PART ONE

Introduction

Chapter One

Introduction

Introduction to Tropical Dermatology

The reader may well ask why we have written another book on tropical dermatology, when at least two good ones currently exist[1,2] and two others could be useful to dermatologists.[3,4] Are there not already too many books on various subjects related to dermatology? Why should two dermatologists working on opposite sides of the world undertake this apparently unnecessary task?

We have felt for some time that practical advice on the diagnosis and handling of tropical dermatoses in a book telling the reader what to do and how to do it in a simple, straightforward way may be more useful than a detailed account of the more highly sophisticated diagnostic procedures that are available in centers of excellence throughout the Western world. Such details are of little practical value to physicians who are seeing patients in the jungles of Africa, in a small mission hospital in South America, in the countryside of Asia, or, for that matter, in any of those areas, where the poverty of the people and of their governments makes it unlikely that they will be able to afford the luxury of recently devised and probably expensive investigations.

In addition, we hope this book will assist not only doctors working in the less sophisticated parts of the world but also those physicians living in the West who find immigrants, refugees, students, and tourists arriving on their doorsteps, bringing with them diseases from elsewhere. Such health care personnel do not need a detailed account of the etiologic or immunologic features of these diseases.

It is not the purpose of this book to be encyclopedic. Out of the innumerable references in the medical literature we have selected and appended to the end of each chapter a small selection of recommended readings for those who wish to expand their knowledge.

In choosing the subjects for this book, we first had to ask ourselves, What is tropical dermatology? Sir Patrick Manson gave an answer many years ago:

"I employ the term 'tropical' in a meteorologic rather than a geographic sense, meaning by it a sustained high atmospheric temperature; and by the term 'tropical diseases,' I wish to indicate diseases occurring only, or which from one circumstance or another are especially prevalent, in warm climates."[5] We are not completely convinced by this definition and believe that on some occasions the word *tropical* is indeed interchangeable with *geographical*—some diseases are limited to certain parts of the world for overt or covert reasons, while others take on different manifestations depending on humidity, sanitation, or the local flora and fauna.

If we were to limit ourselves to the discussion of those problems seen only between the tropics of Cancer and Capricorn, we would have had to exclude almost all of the Middle East (including Iran, Iraq, and most of Saudi Arabia), all of Pakistan and Bangladesh, and most of northern India, and the whole of the north African littoral would also be outside our scope. We have, however, included such diseases as anthrax, favus, and those tropical ulcers whose incidence is highest in the dryer desert areas.

We have not forgotten that such conditions as Gilchrist's disease (originally recognized in Baltimore) and the *Mycobacterium ulcerans* infections (first seen not far from Melbourne), although predominantly found in tropical countries, are not excluded from cooler areas; indeed, many of the diseases common in the jungles of South America and Africa may be found in New York, where, for example, amebiasis is a major problem. Because we are convinced that tropical dermatoses may be seen in affluent as well as in developing countries and in major cities as well as in isolated hamlets, we believe that this book may help not only those doctors working near the equator but also those in subtropical and temperate zones.

We have arranged the chapters in four categories that follow the introductory section. Most of part two (bacterial diseases) is devoted to mycobacterial diseases of the skin, leprosy, tuberculosis, and the Buruli ulcer, but we have also included yaws, anthrax, and the other bacterial ulcers seen in warmer climates.

Part three (fungus diseases) starts with discussions of a few dermatophyte infections that are mainly found in the tropics; however, most of this part covers the deeper mycotic infections. Some of these are almost never seen outside the Americas, while others have a wider distribution. In this part, we have also included actinomycosis, the nocardioses, and botryomycosis, all of which were originally thought to be of fungal origin but are now known to be caused by various bacteria. We have bowed to the tradition that permits inclusion of these diseases in the section on mycology.

Part four consists of a number of parasitic diseases that are most frequently seen in Africa, and part five gives an account of some of the noninfective dermatoses found in the warmer parts of the world.

Realizing as we do that most of our readers will have had little experience in investigating the diseases mentioned here, we have thought it helpful to describe in appendix one certain techniques that may be useful, and in appendix two we list a number of addresses from which may be obtained supplies of those drugs, sera, and laboratory aids that can be more than usually difficult to find.

References

1. Cañizares, O: *Clinical Tropical Dermatology*. London, Blackwell Scientific Publications, 1975.
2. Cañizares, O: *A Manual of Dermatology for Developing Countries*. New York, Oxford University Press, 1982.
3. Maegraith, B: *Adams and Maegraith: Clinical Tropical Diseases*. London, Blackwell Scientific Publications, 1980.
4. Peters, W, Gilles, HM: *Color Atlas of Tropical Medicine and Parasitology*. Chicago, Year Book Medical Publishers, 1977.
5. Manson, P: *Tropical Diseases: A Manual of the Diseases of Warm Climates*. London, Cassell, 1898, p 3.

CHAPTER 2

Clinical Index

Writers and publishers assume that an index is essential, if a medical textbook is to be of real value to its readers. Unfortunately, this is not always true. A typical index, such as the one at the end of this book, is only of use if the reader knows the name of the condition, about which he or she wishes to read. The majority of doctors who, for the first time, see in their clinical practice a case of porokeratosis of Mibelli or lichen sclerosus et atrophicus will, if they do not know its name, be reduced to an aimless leafing through the pages in the hope that the volume will include a photograph that looks something like the condition they have just seen on their patient. If a photograph is not present, the reader may be compelled to read the entire text before realizing that the disease in question is not included.

In a volume such as this, which treats conditions that are rare in many parts of the world, we suspect that most of our readers will not be able instantly to recognize the diseases described and so will not know what to look up in the index.

To help such readers, we have incorporated a clinical index that covers the major clinical presentations (signs, symptoms, and sites) the condition may show. It is *not* an index of all the diseases that show these signs and symptoms but merely a checklist of the major findings of the diseases described here. It is necessarily incomplete—most diseases sometimes occur in unusual presentations and in unexpected sites, and such variants are not included. Similarly, all methods of describing each sign cannot be covered. We believe, however, that if readers list the major features of the case they are trying to diagnose and look them up here, they may well be reminded to add one or two of the more common tropical dermatoses to their list of diagnostic possibilities.

A

Abdomen, abscess	Amebiasis, dracunculosis
distension	Amebiasis, kala-azar
Abscess, epidermal	Botryomycosis, chromomycosis
internal	Amebiasis, dracunculosis
micro-	North American blastomycosis
Achromia	See hypopigmentation
Alopecia	Favus, leprosy, mepacrine eruption
cicatricial	Favus
eyebrows	Anergic leishmaniasis, lepromatous leprosy
Anemia	Kwashiorkor, marasmus, schistosomiasis
Anesthesia of lesions	Leprosy
Animals, spread from	Anthrax, toxoplasmosis
Ankle, papule	Dracunculosis
ulcer	Buruli ulcer
Annular lesions	Borderline leprosy
face	Leprosy
Anus	Amebiasis, mucocutaneous leishmaniasis
Arms	Anthrax, Lobo's disease, pellagra, sporotrichosis
Arthritis, painful	Scurvy
Ascites	Kwashiorkor, leprosy (ENL)
Atrophy of skin	Lupoid leishmaniasis onchocerciasis

B

Bite, insect	Leishmaniasis
Bitot's spots	Kwashiorkor, vitamin A deficiency
Blindness	Onchocerciasis
night	Phrynoderma
Boil, blind	Acute leishmaniasis, anthrax
Bone swelling	See osteomyelitis
pain	Yaws
Bowen's disease	Arsenism
Bulla, multiple	Brazilian pemphigus
single	Dracunculosis
Buttock, nodule	Onchocerciasis
ulcer	Buruli ulcer
verrucous formation	Tuberculosis verrucosa cutis

C

Carcinoma of skin	See epithelioma
Cataract	Onchocerciasis
Cheilitis	Ariboflavinosis, pellagra
Chest wall, edema	Anthrax
sinus	Actinomycosis
vesicles	Brazilian pemphigus
Chiggers	Schistosomiasis
Chorioretinitis	Toxoplasmosis
Chyluria	Filariasis
Cirrhosis	Amebiasis, schistosomiasis
Comedo	Phrynoderma
Condyloma lata	Rhinosporidiosis, yaws
Conjunctivitis	Onchocerciasis
Crusting papules on leg	Schistosomiasis
scalp	Brazilian pemphigus, favus
Cutis laxa	Onchocerciasis

D

Dandruff	Brazilian pemphigus, favus
Dementia	Pellagra
Depression	Pellagra
Dermatitis	Onchoceriasis, schistosomiasis
Diarrhea	Amebiasis, pellagra, phrynoderma, schistosomiasis

E

Ear, nodules	Leishmaniasis, leprosy
erosion	Chiclero ulcer
Earlobe, enlarged	Leprosy
Ecchymoses	Scurvy
Ectropion	Leprosy, North American blastomycosis
Edema	Anthrax, kwashiorkor
of skin	Anthrax
pulmonary	Anthrax
Elbow, ulcer	Buruli ulcer
Elephantiasis	Filariasis
leg	Filariasis
genitalia	Filariasis, schistosomiasis
Encephalitis	Toxoplasmosis
Eosinophilia	Filariasis, dracunculosis, onchocerciasis, schistosomiasis
Epistaxis	Anergic leishmaniasis, rhinosporidiosis

Epithelioma, basal cell — Arsenism
  pseudo epitheliomatous hyperplasia — Buruli ulcer, yaws
  squamous cell — Arsenism
Erosion — See ear, erosion
Erysipelas, bullous — Anthrax
  pseudo — Onchocerciasis
Erythema — Brazilian pemphigus
  febrile — Leprosy (ENL)
  morbilliform — Toxoplasmosis
  nodosum — Tuberculosis, North American blastomycosis
  nodular — leprosy (ENL)
  toxic — Toxoplasmosis
Eschar — Anthrax
Eyebrows, missing — Anergic leishmaniasis, leprosy
Eye changes — Leprosy, phrynoderma, vitamin A deficiency, onchocerciasis

F

Face, annular lesions — Leprosy (borderline)
  destruction — Mucocutaneous, leishmaniasis, tuberculosis, yaws
  leonine — Anergic leishmaniasis, lepromatous leprosy, onchocerciasis
  nodules — Leishmaniasis, Lobo's disease, tuberculosis
  scarred — Leishmaniasis, lupus vulgaris
  smoothed — Leprosy
  ulcerated — Anthrax, leishmaniasis
  vesicles — Brazilian pemphigus
Fever — Anthrax, erythema nodosum leprosum, post-kala-azar leishmaniasis, schistosomiasis
Fingers, contracted — Leprosy, yaws
  ulcerated — Leprosy
Fistula — Actinomycosis, botryomycosis, mycetoma, schistosomiasis, tuberculosis
Follicular plugging — Phrynoderma
Foot, anesthetic — Leprosy
  dropped foot — Leprosy
  infected nodules — Botryomycosis, sporotrichosis

sinuses	Mycetoma, sporotrichosis
mossy	See lymphostasis verrucosa
ulcer	Buruli ulcer, leprosy
Fungus ray	Actinomycosis

G

Gastrointestinal disease	Amebiasis, paracoccidioidomycosis, anthrax
Grains	See granules
Granules, grapelike	Botryomycosis
hard	Mycetoma
in pus	Actinomycosis, botryomycosis, chromomycosis, mycetoma, nocardiosis
soft	Actinomycosis, botryomycosis
yellow	Actinomycosis, botryomycosis, mycetoma
Granuloma	Chromomycosis, leprosy, Lobo's disease, paracoccidioidomycosis, schistosomiasis, tuberculosis
atrophic	Lupoid leishmaniasis, lupus vulgaris, North American blastomycosis
infected	Chromomycosis, schistosomiasis
midline	Mucocutaneous leishmaniasis
mulberry	Paracoccidioidomycosis
nasal	*Mucocutaneous leishmaniasis,* rhinoscleroma, rhinosporidiosis
tuberculoid	Chromomycosis, leishmaniasis, leprosy, tuberculosis
Gumma	Yaws
Gums, bleeding	Ariboflavinosis, scurvy
erosions	Paracoccidioidomycosis

H

Hairs, broken	Favus
fluorescent	Favus
corkscrew	Scurvy
dyschromic	Kwashiorkor
Halo, hypopigmented	Subtropical lichen planus
Hands, crusting	Anthrax, botryomycosis, sporotrichosis
deformed	Leprosy, yaws

Hematuria	Schistosomiasis
Hemorrhage, perifollicular	Scurvy
Hepatosplenomegaly	Kala-azar, schistosomiasis
Hydrocele	Filariasis, onchocerciasis
Hydrocephalus	Toxoplasmosis
Hyperidrosis, palmar or plantar	Arsenism
Hyperkeratosis, plantar	Yaws, Brazilian pemphigus, arsenism
Hyperpigmentation	Arsenism, Brazilian pemphigus, *pellagra*
palm	Tinea nigra
neck	Tinea nigra, pellagra
mottled	Arsenism, onchocerciasis
sun-precipitated	Pellagra
Hyperplasia, pseudoepitheliomatous	Buruli ulcer, yaws
Hypertrophy of lower limb	Filariasis
genitalia	Filariasis
Hypoesthesia	See anesthesia
Hypopigmentation	Arsenism, leprosy, leishmaniasis, onchocerciasis, yaws

I

Ichthyosis	Leprosy
Iliac crest nodules	Onchocerciasis
Induration, inflammatory	Filariasis
acute	Anthrax, botryomycosis
chronic	Actinomycosis, elephantiasis, mossy foot
Isoniazid therapy, reaction to	Pellagra

J

Joints, achromia	Yaws
ankle	Buruli ulcer, dracunculosis, yaws
painful	Scurvy
swollen	Scurvy, tuberculosis

K

Kala-azar	See leishmaniasis
Keloidal scars	Anergic leishmaniasis, Lobo's disease
Keratitis punctata	Leprosy, onchocerciasis
Keratoacanthoma	Arsenism
Keratomalacia	Kwashiorkor, vitamin A deficiency

Keratoses   Arsenism, phrynoderma
Knee, painful   Scurvy
    swollen   Tuberculosis
    ulcer   Buruli ulcer

L
Langhans' cells   Chromomycosis, leprosy
                                                   (tuberculoid), leishmaniasis
                                                   (lupoid), tuberculosis
Larynx, hypertrophic lesions   Rhinoscleroma, rhinosporidiosis
Leonine facies   Anergic leishmaniasis, leprosy
                                                   (lepromatous) onchocerciasis
Lichenification of skin   Onchocerciasis
Lichenoid eruption   Chloriquine, p-aminosalicylic acid
                                                   (and other drugs), lichen planus
                                                   tropicus
Liver, enlarged   Kala-azar, paracoccidioidomycosis,
                                                   leishmaniasis
Loose skin   Onchocerciasis
Lung   See pulmonary disease
Lymphadenitis   Chromomycosis, filariasis, leprosy
                                                   (ENL), paracoccidiodomycosis,
                                                   sporotrichosis, tuberculosis
Lymphadenopathy   Filariasis, onchocerciasis, pian bois,
                                                   sporotrichosis, tuberculosis
Lymphangitis   Filariasis
Lymphedema   Elephantiasis, filariasis,
                                                   onchocerciasis; see also
                                                   lymphostasis verrucosa
Lymphostasis verrucosa   Chromomycosis, filariasis, leprosy,
                                                   yaws

M
Macules, pruritic   Schistosomiasis
Madarosis   Anergic leishmaniasis, leprosy
Malignancies, internal   Arsenism
    skin   Arsenism, Buruli ulcer, tropical
                                                   ulcer, yaws

Melanodermatitis, lichenoid
    mottled   Arsenism
Melanosis   See hyperpigmentation
Meningitis   Toxoplasmosis

Migratory lesions	Dracunculosis, larva migrans
Mossy foot	See lymphostasis verrucosa
Mouth, granuloma	Paracoccidioidomycosis, rhinosporidiosis
strawberry lesions	Rhinosporidiosi
ulceration	Mucocutaneous leishmaniasis, paracoccidioidomycosis, tuberculosis
Mucous, nasal discharge	Rhinosporidiosis

N

"Necklace"	Pellagra
Nerves, enlarged	Leprosy
Neuritis, peripheral	Phrynoderma
Nodule, apple jelly	Lupoid leishmaniasis, lupus vulgaris
edematous	Filariasis, leprosy reactions
face	Leprosy, leishmaniasis
fluctuant	Actinomycosis
generalized	Anergic leishmaniasis, lepromatous leprosy
hypertrophic	Leishmaniasis, Lobo's disease
inflammatory	Botryomycosis, Buruli ulcer, filariasis
perioral	Leishmaniasis
scarring	Leishmaniasis, tuberculosis
subcutaneous	Onchocerciasis
ulcerated	Anthrax, leishmaniasis, leprosy North American blastomycosis, Buruli ulcer, chromomycosis, lichen planus, Lobo's disease, tuberculosis
Nose, blocked	Anergic leishmaniasis, lepromatous leprosy, rhinoscleroma, rhinosporidiosis
collapsed	Leprosy, *leishmaniasis,* tuberculosis, yaws
intranasal nodules	Leprosy, paracoccidioidomycosis, rhinosporidiosis, rhinoscleroma
septal destruction	Leprosy, mucocutaneous leishmaniasis, rhinoscleroma, tuberculosis, yaws

O

Orchitis   Filariasis, leprosy (ENL)
Osteomyelitis   North American blastomycosis,
                                  Madura foot, mycetoma,
                                  tuberculosis, yaws

P

Pain, in nerves   Leprosy reactions
Palate, granuloma   Paracoccidioidomycosis,
                                  rhinoscleroma, rhinosporidiosis

Palm, pigmented   Tinea nigra
Papilloma, conjunctival   Rhinosporidiosis
  strawberry   Rhinosporidiosis
  warty   Chromomycosis, rhinosporidiosis
Papule, craw   Onchocerciasis
  bullous   Dracunculosis
  erythematous   Leprosy (in reaction), yaws
  follicular plugged   Phryhoderma
  hemorrhagic   Anthrax
  hyperpigmented   Lichen planus tropicus
  hypertrophic   Yaws
  pruritic   Drancunculosis, onchocerciasis
  raspberry   Yaws
  violaceous   Lichen planus tropicus
  warty   Chromomycosis, tuberculosis
                                  verrucosa cutis

Perineum, watering-can   Schistosomiasis
Photodermatotis   See sun-sensitivity
Photophobia   Onchocerciasis
Plaque, anesthetic   Leprosy
Pleural effusion   Leprosy (ENL)
Polyp, conjunctival   Rhinosporidiosis
  strawberry   Rhinosporidiosis
Pruritus   Onchocerciasis, schistosomiasis
Pulmonary disease   North American blastomycosis,
                                  paracoccidiodomycosis, tuberculosis
Purpura   Scurvy, toxoplasmosis
Pus, granules in   See granules
  microabscesses   North American blastomycosis,
                                  sporotrichosis

R

Reaction (reversal)   Anergic leishmaniasis, leprosy
Renal disease   Leprosy, North American
                                  blastomycosis

Rhinitis   Rhinoscleroma, leprosy, yaws
Ringworm   See tinea

S
Scaliness, concentric   Tinea imbricata
  diffuse   Brazilian pemphigus, tinea
                                              imbricata
  scalp   Brazilian pemphigus, favus
Scalp   See alopecia
Scars, atrophic   Leishmaniasis, North American
                                              blastomycosis, tuberculosis, yaws
  hypertrophic   Tuberculosis
Scrotum, swelling   Filariasis
Serology   See VDRL
Shins, nodules   Onchocerciasis
Sinuses   Actinomycosis, botryomycosis,
                                              Madura foot, mycetoma, North
                                              American blastomycosis,
                                              tuberculosis

Skin, dyschromic   Arsenism, kwashiorkor, pellagra
  "flaky paint"   Kwashiorkor
  hanging   Onchocerciasis
  hypochromic   Yaws
Soil, infection from   See vegetation
Sore, crusted   Acute leishmaniasis
  ear   Chiclero's ulcer
  facial   Anthrax, leishmaniasis
  multiple   Pian bois
Spirochaetes   Yaws
Spleen, enlarged   Kala-azar, leprosy (ENL),
                                              paracoccidiodomycosis

Spores, thick-walled   Chromomycosis
  golden   Chromomycosis
  multiple budding   Paracoccidioidomycosis
  in sporangia   Rhinosporidiosis
Sunsensitivity   Pellagra, tropicus lichen planus

T
Thorax, sinus   Actinomycosis
Tibia, bowed   Yaws
Tinea, capitis   Favus
  concentric   Tinea imbricata
  pigmented   Tinea nigra

Trachea, blocked	Rhinosporidiosis
Trunk, dyschromic	Arsenism

U

Ulcer	Actinomycosis, botryomycosis, Buruli ulcer, anthrax, amebiasis, diphtheritic ulcer, leprosy, North American blastomycosis, paracoccidiodomycosis, tropical, tropicaloid, tuberculosis
anal	Amebiasis, mucocutaneous leishmaniasis
hemorrhagic	Anthrax
mouth	Paracoccidiodomycosis
nose	Leishmaniasis, paracoccidiodomycosis
penile	North American blastomycosis
phagedenic	Tropical ulcer
plantar	Leprosy
undermined	Buruli ulcer
Umbilicus, granuloma	Schistosomiasis
Urticaria	Dracunculosis, filariasis, schistosomiasis

V

VDRL reactive	Leprosy (Lepromatous), yaws
Vegetation, infection from	Chromomycosis, North American blastomycosis, sporotrichosis
Verrucous formation	Arsenism, chromomycosis, leishmaniasis, tuberculosis verrucosa cutis
Vesicles	Brazilian pemphigus
hemorrhagic	Anthrax
Vincent's organisms	Tropical ulcer
Vitiligo	Onchocerciasis, yaws
Vulva, hypertrophy	Filariasis
ulcer	Amebiasis, mucocutaneous leishmaniasis

W

Weight loss	Kwashiorkor, marasmus, scurvy
Wood, infection from	See vegetation
Wool, infection from	Anthrax

Worm, in deep tissues	Dracunculosis, onchocerciasis, filariasis, schistosomiasis
in eye	Onchocerciasis
in skin	Dracunculosis
Wrist, achromia	Yaws
dropped	Beriberi, leprosy
ulcer	Buruli ulcer, tuberculosis

PART TWO

Bacterial Diseases

CHAPTER 3

Anthrax

Anthrax occurs naturally in herbivorous animals feeding on infected pastures in the dryer parts of the world. Carnivorous animals acquire the infection indirectly by eating infected carcasses of sheep, goats, cows, or even horses, while the disease spreads to humans from contaminated animal products, such as hides, wool or bone meal.

Most commonly seen in the Middle East (especially Iran), not unusual in North or central Africa, central India, and the more arid parts of South America, the condition most frequently affects slaughterers, tanners, skinners, and wool-sorters, as well as others whose occupations bring them into direct contact with animals. In nonendemic areas, infection can be acquired from bone meal, shaving brushes (infected bristles), skins, or raw wool. It has even been reported as spreading from person to person following the communal use of an infected loofah in public baths. The disease may start in any country in the world, although it is more common in the veldt and savannah.

Etiology

The causative organism, *Bacillus anthracis,* is a large Gram-positive organism ($2.5 \mu \times 10–12 \mu$) that occurs singly or in pairs in infected living tissue. It is often difficult to detect these bacilli in the crusted lesions; they can more easily be found by probing the edge of the lesion with a small dental burr using the Dutz technique (see Appendix one).

The organisms produce three different toxins: an edema factor, a protective antigen, and a lethal factor. Different combinations of these three are responsible for the varying pathogenicity of individual strains. When the host animal dies, sporulation takes place; the dormant spores are some of the most resistant living organisms and are known to withstand dry heat at 140°C for more than two hours.

For more than 100 years, it has been known that meat-fed rats are less susceptible to infection than their grain-fed littermates. There is no doubt that human disease is more common in patients with relative protein deficiency, but the major epidemic of inhalation anthrax that occurred a few years ago in Russia shows that even well-fed individuals are susceptible to massive infection.

Clinical Features

Cutaneous Anthrax

The name *malignant pustule* has nothing to recommend it other than tradition because the *B. anthracis* does not stimulate a polymorphonuclear leukocytic reaction. Instead, it causes various types of necrotic lesions, according to the toxicity and virulence of the bacillus.

The mildest form of anthrax starts as a small hemorrhagic papule (Figure 3-1) that is raised and pruritic and rapidly dries up producing a thick necrotic eschar (Figure 3-2), usually on the face or hands, which normally heals without leaving a scar. This type of disease probably occurs in endemic areas fairly frequently without the patients seeking medical assistance.

If the organism is one of the more toxic forms, edema soon supervenes and complicates the ulcer (Figure 3-3). The initial hemorrhagic papule starts to look like a boil or even bullous erysipelas. The lesion becomes surrounded with

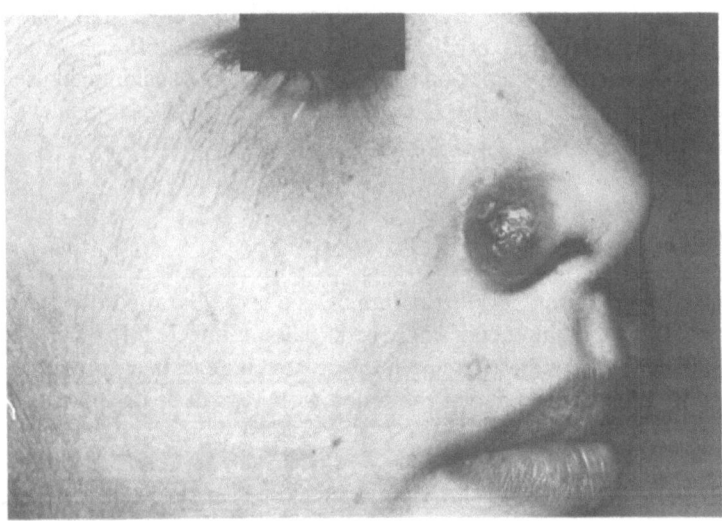

FIGURE 3-1   Hemmorhagic papule with surrounding erythema. (Courtesy Efriede Kohout-Dutz, M.D. and Werner Dutz, M.D., Richmond, Virginia.)

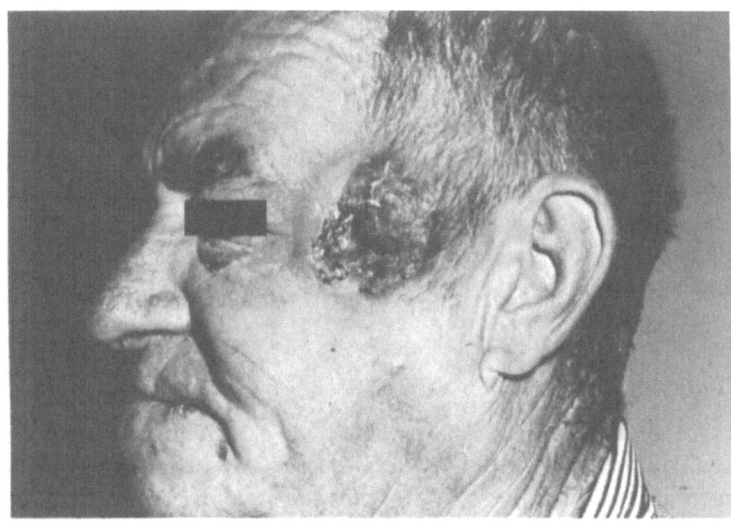

FIGURE 3-2   Thickening and crusting with some necrosis. (Courtesy Efriede Kohout-Dutz, M.D. and Werner Dutz, M.D., Richmond, Virginia.)

hemorrhagic vesicles, and the severe edema may produce an extensive subcutaneous thickening that can be several centimeters thick. Occasionally, severe infections spread along the lymphatics and cause large swellings of regional nodes, but usually the cutaneous lesions remain fairly localized, with a necrotic and hemorrhagic eschar that is surprisingly painless.

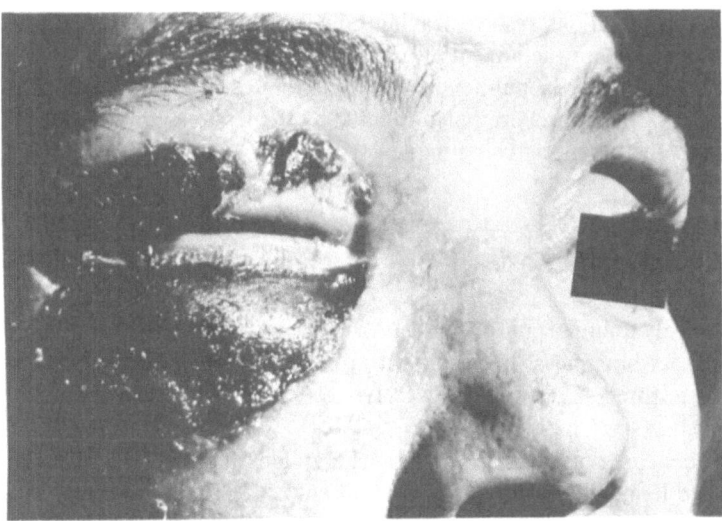

FIGURE 3-3   Edematous thickening of periorbital area with ulceration. (Courtesy Efriede Kohout-Dutz, M.D. and Werner Dutz, M.D., Richmond, Virginia.)

Pulmonary Anthrax

The inhalation of spores most commonly occurs in those who work with treated wool (Osler pointed out nearly a century ago that greasy wool was less dangerous than wool that had been degreased). After they are inhaled, the spores are phagocytosed in the lung tissue and taken to the pulmonary nodes, where they often cause such extreme hemorrhagic lymphadenopathy that the nodes have been described as looking like bags of blood.

Pulmonary edema and septicemia are shortly followed by suffocation and death due to toxemia.

Gastrointestinal Anthrax

This type of anthrax may be acquired by eating contaminated animals. Although a number of cases have been reported with ulceration and edema of the gastrointestinal tract leading to ascites and a profuse watery diarrhea, most cases probably are relatively mild and pass unnoticed in animals and humans.

Natural History

Itching occurs only a few hours after inoculation has taken place, shortly followed by a papulovesicle that crusts to form an eschar. The surrounding tissue may swell severely. If the edema occurs on the hand or arm, relatively little trouble is caused; however, if the edema affects the head and neck, vision, swallowing, or breathing can be greatly hindered. Whereas nowadays the majority of these complications resolve leaving only a scar, some 20 percent of such patients died, before the advent of antibiotics.

Although untreated pulmonary and gastrointestinal infections are often fatal, most patients (and animals) affected by the less toxic organisms get better without the diagnosis being made.

Differential Diagnosis

The relatively unimportant dry eschars sometimes look like an established case of dermal leishmaniasis, but the natural history enables differentiation to be made, as anthrax takes only a few days to develop while leishmaniasis takes much longer (see Chapter 20).

In severe cases of anthrax, the lesions may look like boils or burns, but the edema and hemorrhage are so typical that clinical diagnosis is rarely in doubt. Any suspected case can easily be confirmed by demonstration of organisms in the fluid of the bullae or in nonnecrotic tissue.

Investigations

These large Gram-positive organisms may be confused with *Bacillus cereus* (a nonpathogenic organism of much the same appearance), but if the organism is cultured the characteristic box-car chain of *B. anthracis* will soon develop, and if it is stabbed into gelatin, the typical inverted fir tree can soon be demonstrated.

As most cases of anthrax are easily recognizable, there is little need for histologic study. Biopsies are rarely taken and infrequently helpful. There are no diagnostic histopathologic findings—various combinations of edema, hemorrhage, and necrosis are all that can be seen.

Treatment

The organism seems to be regularly and reliably susceptible to penicillin: penicillin G 600,000 units intramuscularly twice daily for five days or amoxicillin 500 mg every six hours for one week. For patients who are known to be sensitive to penicillin, tetracycline (500 mg every four hours) is also said to be curative.

Under successful treatment, the ulcers heal and the eschars dry up and separate from the underlying skin. Unfortunately, elimination of the *B. anthracis* does not alone save the life of the patients in a more toxic condition; the edema can cause such severe fluid loss that fluid replacement and correction of the electrolyte imbalance may be needed, while toxemia (which is often exacerbated after bacterial death and the subsequent release of further endotoxins) may require heavy doses of corticosteroids for several days.

A vaccine is available in some countries for people who are regularly exposed to infection (see appendix two for addresses), and the suppliers will give recommendations for suitable dosages.

Follow-up

As with all infectious disease, attempts should be made to trace and eliminate sources of infection. Possibly infected hides, skins, hairs, bristles, meats, and bonemeal should be destroyed. Because of the resistant spores that develop in infected carcases, the bodies of animals known to have anthrax should be burned or buried in quicklime. Regrettably, in endemic areas too much pastureland is infected by the spores to make it possible to eradicate the disease in the foreseeable future.

Selected Readings

Amidi, S, Dutz, W, Kohout, E, Ronaghy, HA: Anthrax in Iran. *Z Tropenmed Parasitol* 1977; 24:250.

Davies, JCA: A major epidemic of anthrax in Zimbabwe. *Cent Afr J Med* 1983; 28:291.

Dutz, W: Anthrax, in Braude, AI (ed), *Medical Microbiology and Infectious Disease,* Philadelphia, WB Saunders, 1981, p 1806.

Dutz, W, Kohout-Dutz, E: Anthrax. *Int J Dermatol* 1981; 20:203.

Knight, AH, Wynne-Williams, CJE, Willis, AT: Cutaneous anthrax: The non-industrial hazard. *Br Med J* 1969; 1:416.

Perl, D, Dooley, J: Anthrax, in Binford, CH, Conno, DH (eds), *Pathology of Tropical and Extraordinary Diseases.* Washington, DC, Armed Forces Institute of Pathology, 1976, pp 118–123.

Chapter 4

Yaws

Yaws used to be an extremely common disease in the tropical parts of the world, with millions of cases spreading from the West Indies to the coastal and riverine areas of Central and South America, across the whole of central Africa to Sri Lanka, southern India, Southeast Asia, northern Australia, New Guinea, and the Pacific islands. At one time, it appeared in Scotland as sibbens or the Scottish yaws. Widespread eradication campaigns by WHO and UNICEF during the 1950s were so successful that many authorities believed the disease to be almost extinct. Throughout the 1970s, however, the condition slowly but surely returned to its original homelands.

Patients are usually found among scantily clothed, younger members of the rural population living in high year-round temperatures and humidity, but doctors in temperate zones should not be surprised if an occasional early case (in a refugee or an immigrant) is found in Europe or North America. Scarring and bone deformity associated with the later stages of yaws are more likely to be seen outside endemic areas and can pose diagnostic problems.

Etiology

Yaws is one of the diseases caused by a spirochete. There is considerable debate about the *Treponema pertenue*. Scattered throughout the world is a range of treponematoses: venereal syphilis, bejel, pinta, and yaws are the most extensive. Although these diseases have such varied clinical presentations, the causative organisms seem to be undifferentiable, and there is disagreement as to whether the *T. pallidum* (syphilis, bejel), the *T. carateum* (pinta), and the *T. pertenue* (yaws) are indeed separate organisms. Clinically, however, there is no doubt that yaws is a separate disease whose signs and symptoms differ from those of the other trepanematoses.

It is transmitted by skin-to-skin nonvenereal contact and usually starts on uncovered sites in children, where bites, scratches, and grazes facilitate bacterial penetration of the epidermis.

The inability of the spirochete to grow in culture has made it impossible to search for it outside the human body, and it is not known whether *T. pertenue* confines itself to humans or whether it can exist elsewhere; its very slow return from almost complete eradication suggests that there are no major sources of infection outside humankind and that person-to-person contact is the only mode of transmission.

Clinical Features

In the past, it was the custom to divide the clinical features of yaws into primary, secondary, and tertiary lesions (perhaps encouraged by comparison with the clinical features of syphilis), but it is simpler to group the primary and secondary lesions together, as they tend to overlap and are separated by a period of latency from those forms previously called tertiary.

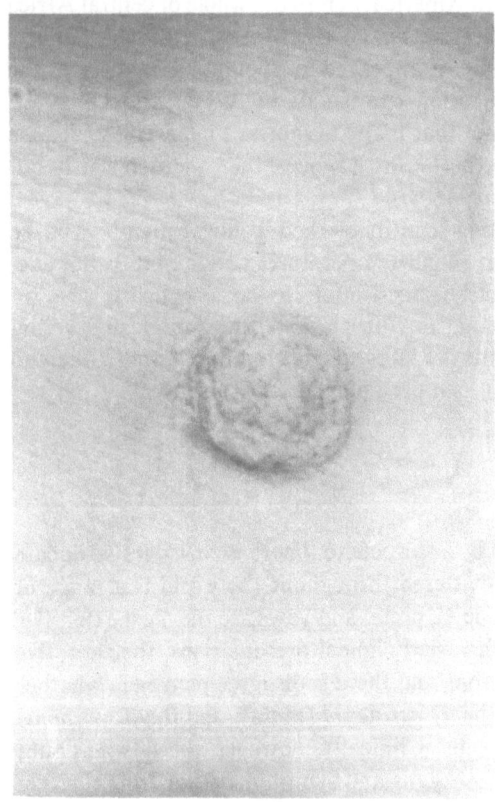

FIGURE 4-1 Mother yaw: small crusted papillomatous lesion. (Courtesy Arturo Tapia, M.D., Panama City, Panama.)

Early Yaws

The initial lesion, often known as the mother yaw (Figure 4-1), starts as a small erythematous papule, enlarges to give a proliferating and crusting papilloma, spreads and ulcerates for two to six months (sometimes even longer), and finally heals spontaneously, leaving a large depressed scar.

The features that used to be called secondary are manifestations of the blood-borne spread of infection. Waves of skin lesions erupt, often associated with severe bone pain caused by periostitis and with swelling of the joints of the legs, hands, and feet.

The skin conditions are basically of two types, the papular and the hyperkeratotic. Soft proliferating papules looking like raspberries (hence the name *frambesia*) (Figures 4-2, 4-3) start to break out well before the disappearance of the mother yaw. Called daughter yaws, these differ from the original patch only in size and not in nature; they erupt in crops all over the body, proliferating, oozing, healing, and recurring for two or three years. They rarely ulcerate and do not leave scars. If the mucous membranes are affected (the mouth and perineum in particular), the papillomata take the form of soft, moist condylomata lata.

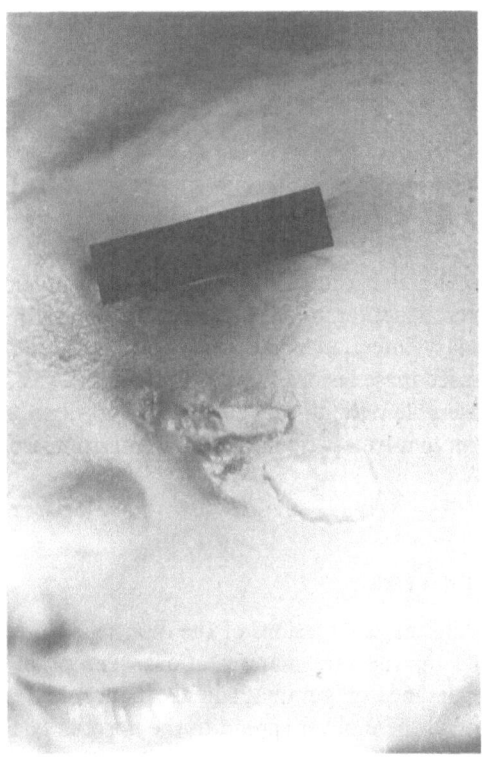

FIGURE 4-2 Frambesia: soft proliferating papules. (Courtesy Arturo Tapia, M.D., Panama City, Panama.)

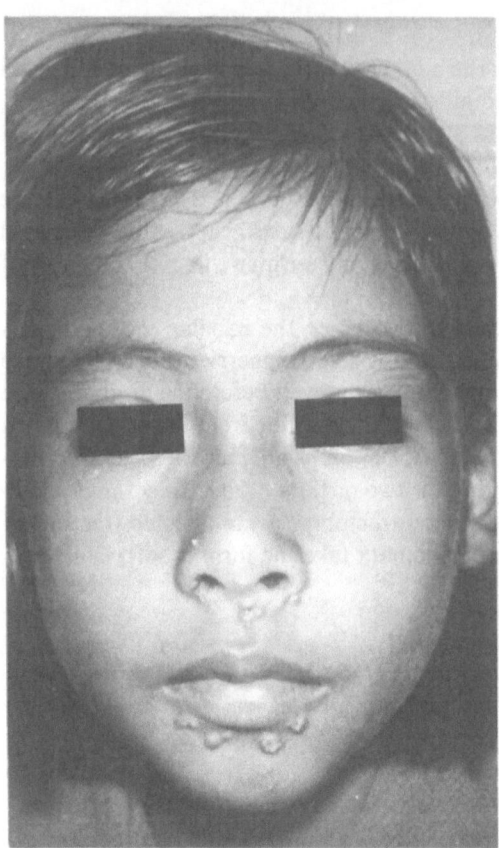

FIGURE 4-3 Verrucous secondary lesions. (Courtesy D. Ngreh, M.D., Penang, Malaysia.)

Although the palms and soles may develop typical wet papillomata, more often hyperkeratotic patches form especially on the soles. Fissuring and secondary infection make walking painful and cause the typical gait that has caused these lesions to be known as crab yaws. Early yaws finally subsides; the miserable patient, relieved of the sores and bone pain, enters into a relatively symptom-free period of latency interrupted only by occasional attacks of crab yaws.

Late Yaws

While the early lesions of the disease are rarely destructive, this does not hold true for the late manifestations. The onset of late yaws is marked by the appearance of gummata in the bone, skin, and subcutaneous tissues. Fortunately, these never spread to the nervous system or the cardiovascular system.

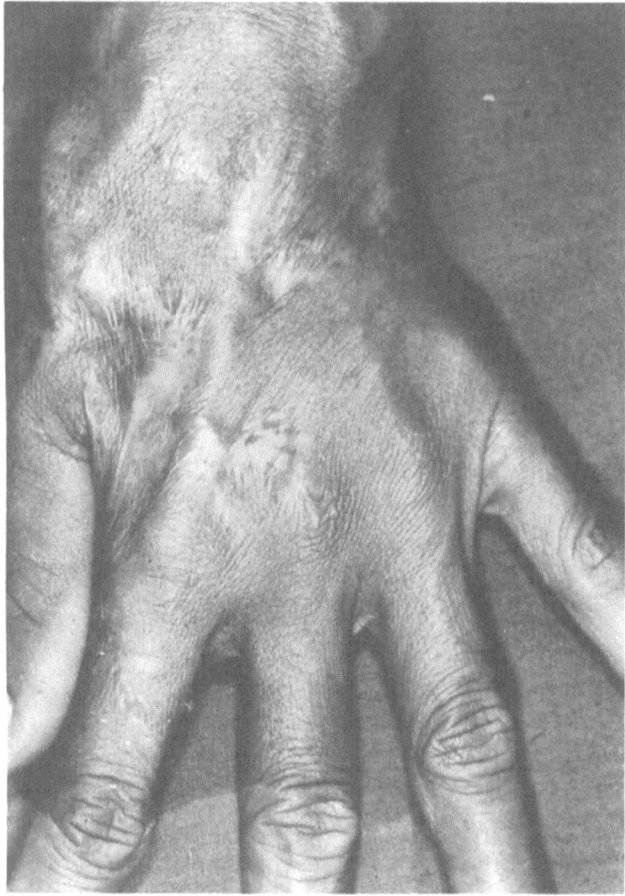

FIGURE 4-4   Scarring and distortion from late yaws.

Gummatous osteitis and periostitis cause severe bone pain and may result in hypertrophy or necrosis. A sabre tibia shows anterior bowing and thickening, nodular swelling of the skull causes frontal bossing and swelling, and necrosis of the carpal bones may lead to destruction of the wrist (Figure 4-4). Particularly in Africa, the center of the face may collapse following destruction of the nasal septum (gangosa) (Figure 4-5). Hypertrophy of the maxillae, known as goundou, is sometimes attributed to yaws.

In the skin, the gumma starts as a nodule that enlarges and breaks down in the center to cause a punched-out ulcer that slowly heals, leaving a thin, wrinkled, tissue-paper scar. This process may take years, during which neighboring lesions may coalesce to produce serpiginous ulcers, which, if combined with

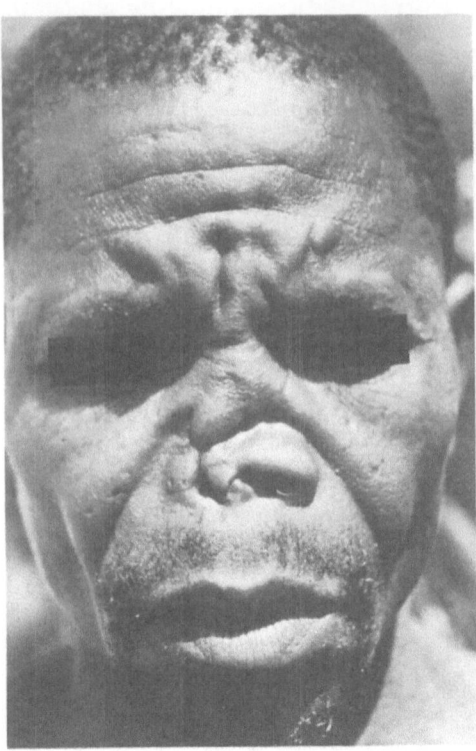

FIGURE 4-5 Gangosa: inactive late yaws. (Courtesy Liverpool School of Tropical Medicine.)

underlying bone or joint disease, may cause severe deformity and even produce elephantiasis in the distal part of the affected limb.

Browne points out that certain areas—the triangular area on the anterior aspect of the wrist, the shin, and the fronts of elbows and ankles—may show a depigmentation amounting to complete achromia. If this is present, it is strong confirmatory evidence that associated chronic ulcerated or scarring lesions are caused by late yaws rather than syphilis or tuberculosis.

Epitheliomatous change has been known to complicate these ulcers or their succeeding scars.

Natural History

The mother yaw appears some two to six weeks after initial infection; it is unlikely that the disease ever undergoes spontaneous cure, although with time, each individual lesion may resolve. In the early period, the lesions are predominantly soft papillomatous excrescences that, except for the mother yaw, do not scar (Figure 4-6). This period may last for up to five years, after which a five-

FIGURE 4-6 Active yaws with multiple soft papillomata and postinflammatory pigmentation. (Courtesy Liverpool School of Tropical Medicine.)

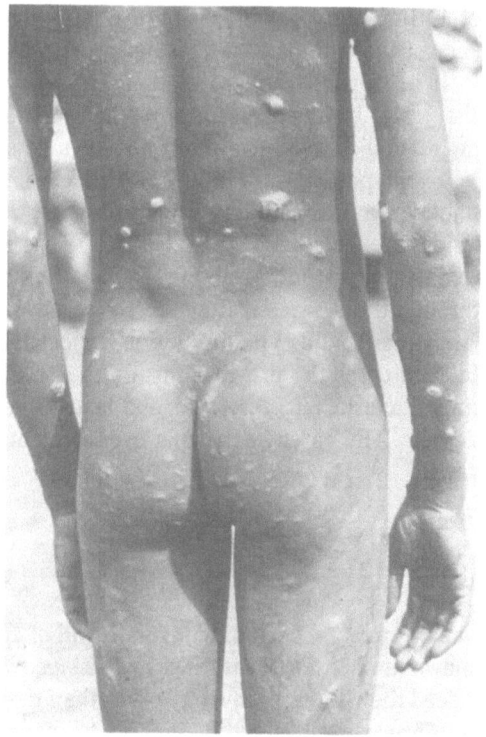

to ten-year period of latency occurs, followed by the appearance of gummatous lesions.

The only dermatologic link between these two active periods is seen on the palms and soles, where patches of hyperkeratosis, nodular or flat, fissured and painful, may come and go, causing few symptoms other than a painful hindrance to walking.

When the late lesions appear, they will probably continue to cause trouble until treatment is undertaken. Although individual lesions slowly regress, the ulceration and bone deformities can be expected to last indefinitely.

Differential Diagnosis

Because of the long period during which yaws seemed almost entirely to have disappeared, its recent resurgence has often taken the medical profession by surprise, and the diagnosis, at least in the early stages, has frequently been missed. The mother yaw can be differentiated from the ulcerative proliferation of anthrax by the absence of complicating edema, plus the malignant pustule

of anthrax develops much more rapidly than yaws and the geographic indic-
ence of the two diseases does not overlap at all.

In the eruptive phase of daughter yaws, the raspberry-shaped papilloma
should not be mistaken for any other condition, while condylomata around the
mouth and anus almost never appear unless in association with other signs.

The hyperkeratotic lesions of the feet and hands should be easily differentiable from palma-plantar keratoses not only because of the history (such
lesions are usually congenital or familial), but also because these rather localized hyperkeratotic swellings of yaws often ooze a spirochete-containing serum
through the fissures if they are squeezed. It is sometimes difficult to separate
late yaws from a syphilitic lesion, especially a syphilitic plantar keratoderma.
In such cases the previous history is almost the only helpful clinical feature,
since bacteriologic, serologic, and histopathologic investigations are of very little help. The patchy achromia over some of the joints may be a useful clue to
yaws.

Investigations

In early yaws, the exuding serum is full of spirochetes. As there is no presently
known method for separating *T. pertenue* from *T. pallidum* or *T. carateum* (if
indeed they differ in any way other than tissue preference and virulence), finding an organism is rarely the aid to diagnosis that might be expected. The
clinical appearance is more reliable because the mother yaw is larger, softer,
and longer-lasting than a syphilitic chancre. It usually develops on the exposed
parts of the limbs or face.

All the serologic tests used for syphilis are also positive for *T. pertenue.*
These investigations are of no help in differentiating the two conditions.

If a gumma is biopsied, it is frequently indistinguishable from syphilis—all
cases of syphilis and yaws show heavy plasma-cell infiltrates. It has been
pointed out that the histology of the early lesions may show two helpful features. The endarterial proliferation common in syphilis is absent in yaws, and
sometimes in yaws there is a profuse invasion of spirochetes into the epidermis.
This is the only real differentiation from syphilis, in which the organisms are
mesodermotropic and are not found in the epidermis in significant numbers.

Treatment

Twenty-five years ago, it was believed that penicillin was curative and that a
single injection of 1.2 million units of penicillin G was all that was needed to
eradicate the disease in an adult. Newly seen cases are as susceptible as other's
to a single injection, but the disease must have returned either because infection spread into the treated area from elsewhere or, equally possible and more

worrisome, treatment did not eradicate all the organisms in every patient. It is urged that 1.2 million units of penicillin G be injected into each buttock of the patient and all the immediate contacts: the previously recommended half-dose for contacts is not recommended.

If a patient is sensitive to penicillin, large doses of tetracycline or erythromycin (2 g daily for two weeks) may be substituted.

Selected Readings

Browne, SJ: Yaws. *Br Med J* 1980; 281:1090.

Browne, SJ: Yaws. *Int J Dermatol* 1982; 21:220.

Endemic treponematoses in the 1980's. *Lancet* 1983; 2:552.

Hackett, CJ: Yaws. WHO monograph series No. 36, 1957.

Hackett, CJ, Guthe, T: Yaws. *Bull WHO* 1956; 15:869.

Lanigan-O'Keefe, FM, Holmes, JG, Hill, D: Infectious and active yaws in a Midland city. *Br J Dermatol* 1967; 79:325.

Morton, RS: The sibbens of Scotland. *Med Hist* 1967; 11:374.

Willcox, RR: The treponemal evolution. *Trans St. John's Hosp Dermatol Soc* 1972; 58:21.

Chapter 5

Tuberculosis of the Skin

In the past 40 years, the incidence of tuberculosis has declined steadily throughout the Western world. It is not known whether this is due to the successful use of BCG as an antituberculosis vaccine (a belief widely held in Europe) or whether it is simply the result of a better standard of living and more efficacious antituberculosis therapy (more widely believed in the United States). Tuberculosis is still rife in the less affluent parts of the third world; however, it is not a tropical disease in the same sense as are onchocerciasis and rhinoscleroma. Its high persistance in the tropics justifies the consideration of cutaneous tuberculosis in this book.

Etiology

Three types of *Mycobacterium tuberculosis* known to produce disease in humans (human, bovine, and avian) can enter the human body by inhalation, ingestion or inoculation.

Human tuberculosis (which most commonly affects the skin and the lungs) is transmitted from person to person by droplet infection from the cough of a patient with pulmonary disease or by inhalation of dust contaminated by infected sputum. Bovine tuberculosis is usually acquired from infected milk and affects the gastrointestinal tract and the cervical and abdominal lymph nodes. Little is known about avian tuberculosis except that it is less common and perhaps less sensitive to treatment.

Inoculation is the commonest cause of cutaneous tuberculosis, being found in butchers and slaughterhouse workers whose cuts and grazes can be contaminated by material from infected animals. Surgeons and pathologists may be similarly infected in their professional work. In the tropics, lightly-dressed individuals who are in the habit of sitting on the floor of wooden houses may acquire lesions from an infected splinter. Cutaneous tuberculosis may also result from extension of the disease from an underlying bone, joint, or lymph node.

When the organism enters a person for the first time, the body reacts with a nonspecific inflammation with polymorphonuclear leukocytes and necrosis. This form of reaction is unsuccessful in handling the infection. Within two or three weeks the histology changes and a granulomatous reaction slowly takes over. With the appearance of epithelioid cells, mycobacteria diminish in number; presumably in many patients, this process satisfactorily cures the infection. If the T-cells are not fully competent, differing clinical pictures are found, varying from lupus vulgaris, with high but incomplete immunity via scrofuloderma (moderate immunity), to miliary tuberculosis, in which little or no immunity exists.

Clinical Features

Tuberculous Chancre

This is a rare condition that develops only when intradermal inoculation affects a previously uninfected patient (Figure 5-1). A small, usually painless, nodule containing numerous tubercle bacilli breaks down rapidly, producing a ragged

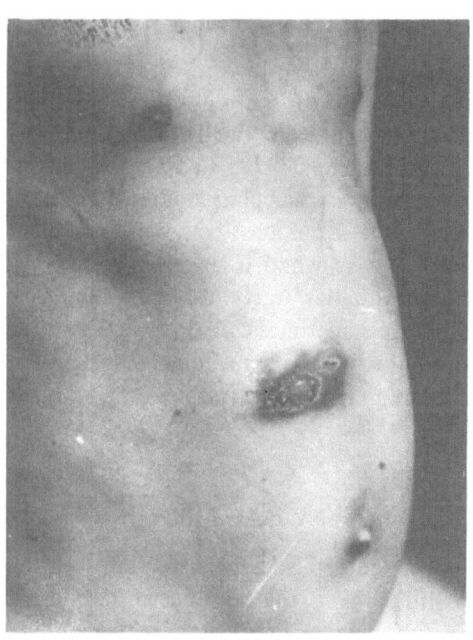

FIGURE 5-1 Tuberculous chancre. (Courtesy Mohsen Soliman, M.D., Cairo, Egypt.)

ulcer covered by a crust. This is followed by enlargement of the regional lymph nodes, which liquefy and discharge. The diagnosis is often not made until a painless unilateral adenitis draws attention to a healing scar.

Scrofuloderma

Scrofuloderma is caused by a liquifying, caseating necrosis extending into and through the skin from underlying disease, usually lymphadenitis or tuberculous osteitis. In almost all cases, there is clinical evidence of the associated abnormality. First, painless bluish-red nodules enlarge and ulcerate. Later, sinuses can be found tracking from the soft underlying tissues, and, finally, an irregularly scarred and fluctuant mass forms that discharges, ulcerates, and heals at the same time around a group of sinuses and fistulae (Figure 5-2).

Tuberculous Ulcers

When infection spreads to the skin from an underlying tuberculous bone or joint (usually the sternum, ribs, hands, wrists, feet, and ankles), the skin soon breaks down, producing an ulcer with a bluish edge. Sometimes an ulcer develops in mucous membranes after autoinoculation from bacilli in the sputum, urine, or feces; these ulcers may spread to the adjacent skin. The clinical appearance is not specific, although the lesion is full of bacilli.

Tuberculosis Verrucosa Cutis

When tuberculosis involves the upper part of the dermis, the epidermis sometimes reacts with a proliferative hyperplasia, and warty nodules develop that slowly extend centrifugally to produce irregular verrucose plaques, often with a central atrophic scar in which further nodules may develop. This happens when bacterial inoculation affects a patient already sensitized to the tubercle bacillus. It is the most common form of tuberculosis of the skin in India and southeast Asia and is usually found on the buttocks or ankles, knees, and elbows. Smaller, warty lesions on the fingers of butchers or postmortem attendants are sometimes called verruca necrogenica. The plaques are often fissured and sometimes have pustules and superficial discharging abscesses to produce a lesion that is boggy rather than warty and often only diagnosed on biopsy (Figure 5-3).

Miliary Tuberculosis

In those deprived areas where pulmonary tuberculosis still poses a major public health problem, it is not unusual to find patients whose physiologic, dietetic, or immunologic deficiencies have permitted the establishment of an engulfing

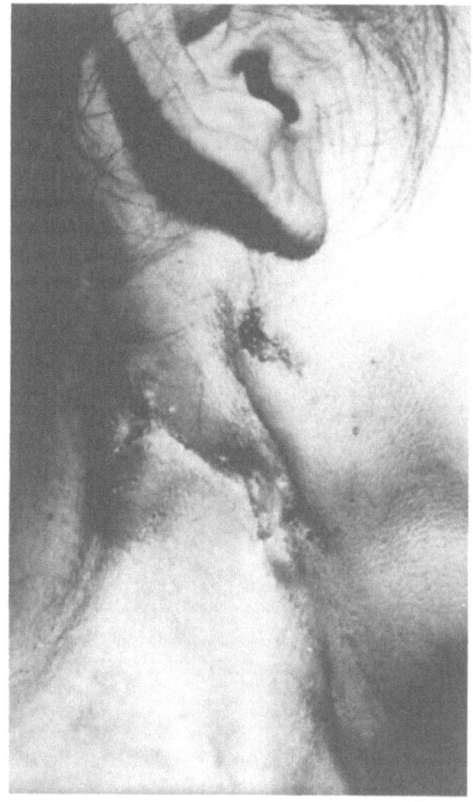

FIGURE 5-2 Scrofuloderma: note ulcerations and fluctuant masses around sinus tracts. (Courtesy Marwali Harahap, M.D., Rumah Sakit Pirngada, Medan, Indonesia, with permission of the *International Journal of Dermatology* and the International Society of Tropical Dermatology.)

infection that permeates the whole body before it kills the patient. The skin is not free from this disaster, and such patients may develop an explosion of papulovesicles. This eruption will usually be recognized only by its association with severe weight loss and the other signs of generalized disease.

Lupus Vulgaris

The most famous form of cutaneous tuberculosis is today less common than tuberculosis verrucosa cutis. Patients whose reaction to a primary infection has protected them for several years will, if reinfected, develop a high immunity tuberculous granuloma. The reinfecting organism may arrive in the skin by primary inoculation or by direct extension: lupus vulgaris can be seen beside a patch of scrofuloderma or breaking out in what was apparently an old tuberculous scar.

A slowly extending plaque develops, studded with many small translucent nodules best demonstrated by diascopy (see appendix one). It has been the

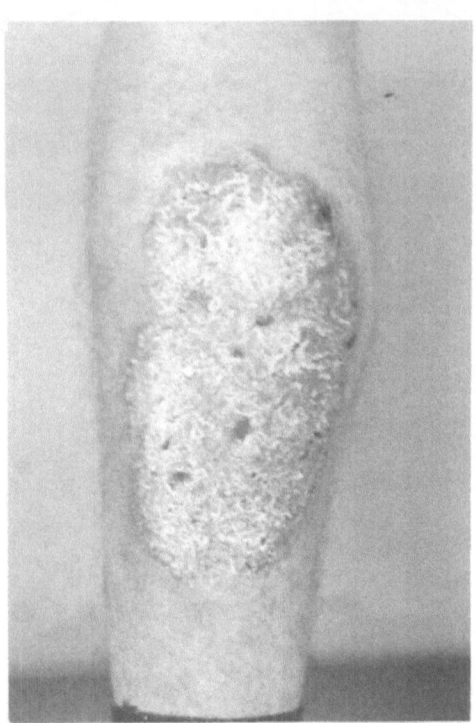

FIGURE 5-3 Tuberculosis verrucosa cutis. Crusting, redness, and scaling on leg. (Courtesy Stephanie Jablonska, M.D., Warsaw, Poland.)

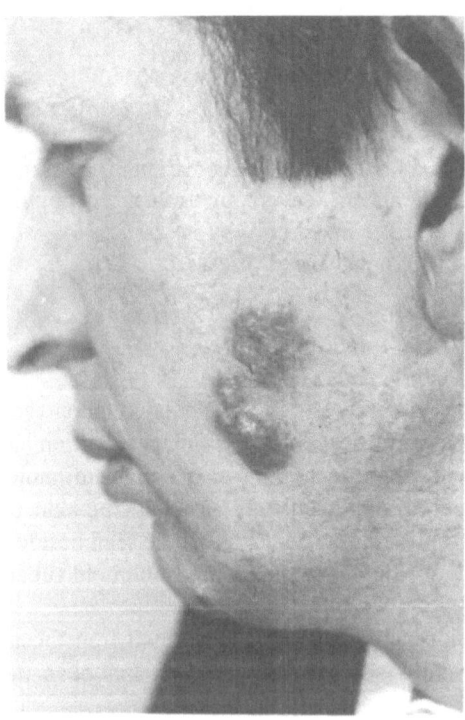

a

FIGURE 5-4 Lupus vulgaris. a. Apple jelly nodules on face. (Courtesy Stephanie Jablonska, M.D., Warsaw, Poland.)

FIGURE 5-4 b. More extensive
lesions with central ulcerations.
(Courtesy Stephanie Jablonska,
M.D., Warsaw, Poland.)

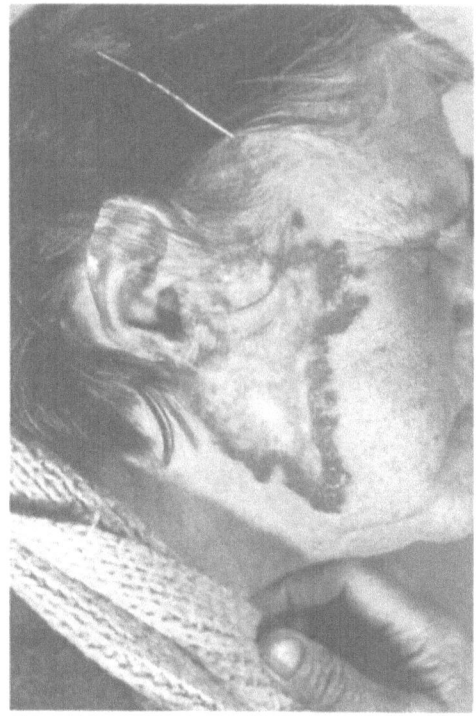

b

habit in the West to call these nodules apple jelly (Figure 5-4a), because they
appear greenish-yellow in Caucasian or oriental skin, but the term is inaccurate
for Africans and Asians, whose nodules are orange-brown. Peripheral expan-
sion will often leave a central scar that can be keloidal but is more often
atrophic with a tendency to ulcerate. It is not unusual for further lupus nodules
to form in the scar (Figures 5-4b, c).

In the past, lupus vulgaris frequently affected the center of the face (hence
the name—the mutilation produced is similar to the damage found in a person
savaged by a wolf). Destruction of the nose and nasal septum can cause the
nose to collapse, producing a parrot beak deformity. Lupus vulgaris produces
a range of clinical changes, from the atrophic and ulcerating to the hypertrophic and pseudotumorous, but in all types the active lupus nodule can be
detected.

Other Tuberculous Lesions

Various other lesions were frequently described in early textbooks as being seen
in patients with tuberculosis. It is now believed that some tuberculids' (erythema induratum, lupus miliaris disseminatus faciei, acne agminata, rosaceous
tuberculid, etc.) are not of tuberculous etiology. Two other conditions are
thought to be true tuberculids: lichen scrofulosorum and papulonecrotic tub-

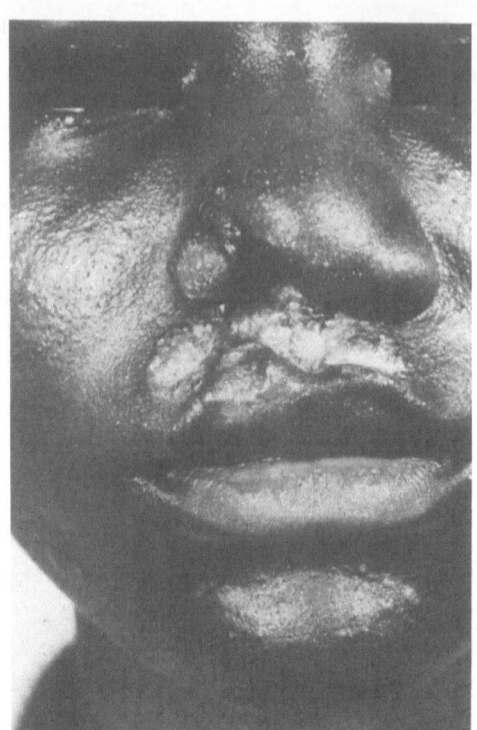

FIGURE 5-4 c. Ulceration and atrophy on upper lip. (Courtesy Marwali Harahap, M.D., Rumah Sakit Pirngada, Medan, Indonesia.)

c

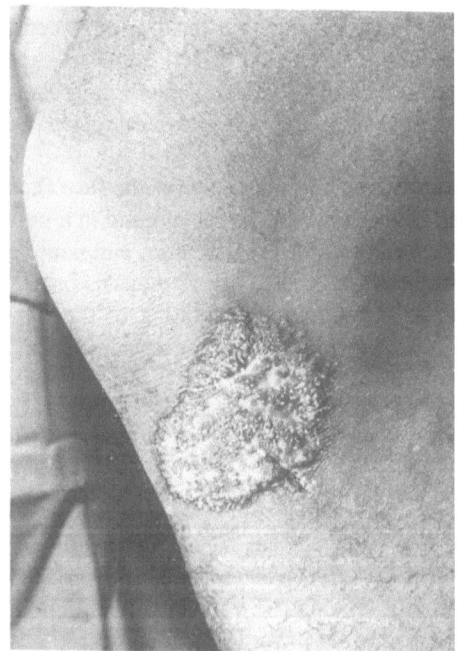

d

FIGURE 5-4 d. Lupus vulgaris below the knee spreading pheripherally. (Courtesy J. Sidney Rice, M.D. Collection of the College of Physicians of Philadelphia.)

erculids are both rare. They show outcrops of lichenoid or centrally necrotic papules and are often difficult to cure.

Natural History

Not every tubercle bacillus that successfully penetrates the human skin will cause a recognizable infection; most people can satisfactorily eliminate the invaders. Patients with an inadequate immune status develop diseases that progress inexorably, with scarring and destruction extending in all directions.

The time between inoculation and the appearance of a tuberculous chancre is only a matter of weeks, but it may be many years before lupus vulgaris appears. The patient shown in Figure 5-3 developed lupus vulgaris in the scar of an operation that had been performed for tuberculous osteitis 47 years previously.

Differential Diagnosis

The acute onset of a small tuberculous chancre that ulcerates and crusts may be confused with an early dry case of anthrax (see chapter 3) and can also be mistaken for the infection caused by *Mycobacterium balnei* (swimming pool or fish tank granuloma), but this only rarely spreads to the regional lymph nodes.

Scrofuloderma can usually be recognized fairly easily. Sporotrichosis involves lymph nodes, where it causes a large discharging inguinal or axillary mass, but it rarely affects cervical nodes, while on the limbs it is possible to find a chain of nodules along the lymphatics connecting the primary lesion with the regional adenopathy. Actinomycosis is easily distinguished by the yellow granules in the discharge.

Tuberculosis verrucosa cutis is easily differentiated from verruca vulgaris when the lesion is larger than 1 cm in diameter. The hyperkeratotic lesions of chromomycosis can have a similar appearance but rarely show atrophy. Syphilitic gummata have a much shorter clinical history—what syphilis does in months, tuberculosis does in years. Hypertrophic lichen planus is usually pruritic, multiple, and limited to the lower limbs. If the patient has been unfortunate enough to acquire an infection by one of the rarer mycobacteria, the diagnosis will never be confirmed unless a bacteriologist can produce a successful and diagnostic culture.

Lupus vulgaris is occasionally mimicked by a patch of tuberculoid leprosy but is of course not anesthetic. In some parts of the world, sarcoidosis, which affects Africans more than Asians, will sometimes show clinically similar lesions, but the Mantoux test is negative. It is most difficult to differentiate between lupus vulgaris and the chronic lupoid form of leishmaniasis (see chapter 20); a careful clinical history may help establish the diagnosis.

Investigations

Bacteriology

The detectable presence of acid-fast bacilli is not diagnostic. *M. leprae, M. ulcerans, M. balnei,* and other atypical mycobacteria can all invade the skin. It may be necessary to take a punch biopsy, extract the organisms, and set up cultures in vitro (Lowenstein-Jensen medium) and in vivo (guinea pig inoculation). It is recognized that the subleties of mouse footpad culture will usually not be available.

In orificial tuberculosis and scrofuloderma and other types where there is an underlying active tuberculosis, suitable investigations may demonstrate mycobacteria in the sputum, gastric washings, or even in the urine or feces. Discharge from the sinuses of scrofuloderma should also be examined.

Histopathology

When a patient is suspected of having tuberculosis of the skin, the most important investigation is a biopsy. Sections should be stained not only with hematoxylin and eosin but also with Ziehl-Neelsen stain to demonstrate acid-fast bacilli.

In a classical tuberculous granuloma, epithelioid cells and some Langhans' giant cells are surrounded by a mantle of lymphocytes. Numerous acid-fast bacilli are found in the primary chancre and scrofuloderma, but these are uncommon in warty tuberculosis and rare or completely absent in lupus vulgaris and the tuberculids. Caseation occurs to some degree in all forms of tuberculosis, being proportional to the number of mycobacteria in the lesions, but unfortunately these granulomata are not diagnostic even in the presence of caseation, which may also be seen in tuberculoid leprosy, particularly the neural form. Tuberculoid granulomata are found not only in leprosy but also in chromomycosis and chronic leishmaniasis. Careful search must be made for distinguishing features. Destruction of small nerves in the skin by a tuberculoid granuloma is evidence of leprosy, while the classical golden-brown spores of chromomycosis are diagnostic. Unfortunately, the Leishman-Donovan body is no more frequently seen in chronic leishmaniasis than is *M. tuberculosis* in lupus vulgaris. Further investigations are needed to determine whether the granuloma is tuberculous or tuberculoid.

Other Tests

Every case of suspected cutaneous tuberculosis should have an x-ray of the chest in case of concomitant pulmonary infection, and erythrocyte sedimentation rate (ESR) should be determined.

The Mantoux test will almost always be positive. If it is negative, further consideration should be given to the possibility that the patient has sarcoidosis, chromomycosis, or lupoid leishmaniasis.

If the diagnosis remains uncertain, it may be necessary to perform a therapeutic trial as a last resort. Patients who do not show definite improvement within two months of the onset of effective therapy do not have skin tuberculosis.

Treatment

When cutaneous tuberculosis is associated with an underlying disease, it is sometimes difficult to decide who should treat the patient. It is recommended that treatment be supervised by a team rather than an individual. If this is not possible, all cases should be treated as if there were active underlying disease. If suitable laboratory facilities are available, drug sensitivity studies should be made to determine which medication should be used. In the absence of such tests the following routine is suggested:

1. Patients should be given 300 mg of isonicotinic acid hydrazide daily in a single dose and rifampin 600 mg daily. Both treatments should be continued for one year after the disappearance of all signs of clinical activity.
2. For diseases with a high bacterial content, ethambutol (not more than 20 mg/kg) should supplement therapy for the first two months in an effort to reduce the bacterial load as quickly as possible. (Ethambutol should not be given to children under six years of age.) All these drugs can be taken in single daily doses—there is no advantage in divided dosage.

Before the development of specific antituberculosis drugs, calciferol was used with success in the treatment of lupus vulgaris. In tropical countries where pulmonary disease is still rampant, the incidence of cutaneous disease is smaller than might be expected. This may be due to the prolonged exposure to sunlight of many of the lightly clad indigenous population, and perhaps this is why most cases of cutaneous tuberculosis resolve spontaneously on monotherapy with isoniazid. The possibility is quite high that the infecting organism may now be resistant to isoniazid, which, combined with the possible coexistence of an underlying infection that has been overlooked, makes it advisable that all patients be treated with polytherapy.

Follow-up

Patients should be seen every two weeks for the first two months of treatment and then at monthly intervals until the lesion has disappeared and treatment has been stopped. It must always be expected that diseases that have healed with atrophy may in the long term undergo malignant degeneration. Patients should be warned that the appearance in a scar of a nodule or an erosion should not go unchecked. Such lesions should be biopsied if there is any doubt as to their nature. It is probably wise for all those with atrophic scars on exposed areas to be protected by sun barriers for the rest of their lives.

Selected Readings

Brown, FS, Anderson, RH, Burnett, JW: Cutaneous tuberculosis. *J Am Acad Dermatol* 1982; 6:101.

Harahap, M: Tuberculosis of the skin. *Int J Dermatol* 1983; 22:542.

Immunological tests for tuberculosis, *Lancet* 1983; 1:1024.

Morrison, JG, Fourie, ED: The papulonecrotic tuberculide—from arthus reaction to lupus vulgaris. *Br J Dermatol* 1974; 91:263.

Ut, NV: Cutaneous tuberculosis in Vietnam. *Int J Dermatol* 1973; 21:372.

Walker, AE, Frenk, E, Smith, AJ: Therapeutics XVII—reserve drugs in the treatment of tuberculosis *Br J Dermatol* 1972; 86:210.

Wardman, AG, Williams, SF, Curzon, PGD, et al: Tuberculosis—who should prescribe? *Br Med J* 1982; 2:569.

CHAPTER 6

Leprosy

No physician should be surprised if the next patient he or she sees has leprosy—it has been found in every country in the world. Variously described as starting in China or India, it is reputed to have been carried to the Middle East and Europe by troops returning from the campaigns of Alexander the Great. The relative lack of medical sophistication in the first half of the Christian era resulted in leprosy being called by many names, and similarly many diseases were called leprosy. Clarification of this confusion has become possible because the bone changes associated with severe untreated disease are now easily recognizable, and studies in cemeteries, catacombs, and other burial places have made it possible to detect whether or not leprosy existed in a certain area at a certain time. Despite the original diagnostic uncertainty, which probably caused the incarceration of many patients who did not actually have the disease, it is now known, for example, that many people buried in the Aebelholt monastery in Denmark between 1175 and 1544 were definitely infected.

The medieval remains found in northern Europe and the fact that the causative organism was originally found by Armauer Hansen in Bergen, working with Norwegian patients, have not prevented the lay public from believing that the disease is limited to tropical countries. It is true that in the past 100 years it has disappeared from Scandinavia and England, while patients now being detected in Japan and the United States have almost always acquired the infection elsewhere. New cases still originate in Spain, Malta, southern Italy, Greece, Turkey, and Cyprus, as well as in the Middle East. Africa, Central and South America, Asia, and the Pacific islands all have leprosy to a greater or lesser extent.

It should be emphasized, however, that the increased mobility of the world's population, traveling voluntarily (tourists, immigrants, and students) or involuntarily (refugees and military personnel), has ensured that, at least sporadically, leprosy can occur everywhere.

Etiology

When the *Mycobacterium leprae* attempts to establish itself in the human body, the clinical picture that develops is not of a unique and diagnostic cluster of signs and symptoms. An astonishing range of different presentations can be seen, from a single enlarged painless nerve or a small localized patch of skin that is anesthetic to a most profuse eruption of shiny nodules covering the whole body and showing no evidence of sensory loss. It is a matter of wonder that physicians working in the past without any knowledge of the pathology or the etiology should have been able to recognize that these widely varying symptom complexes were manifestations of the same disease, more particularly, since in some forms of leprosy, mycobacteria are so few in number that they are usually undetectable, and the widely differing presentations show an enormous difference in their histopatholgy.

Immunologic Background

The different types of leprosy are not caused by varying species of *M. leprae*, but rather by the varying susceptibilities of different individuals. It is probably true that, despite various claims to the contrary, the leprosy bacillus has never been cultured in vitro. We cannot be certain that different varieties of the organism do not exist, but even if that were the case, there is little reason to believe that the body would react differently to such variants.

It is not known how the disease is transmitted; the suggestion in the past of prolonged contact with an infected person is completely untenable. The *M. leprae* may occasionally penetrate the skin after trauma, but more likely leprosy is caused by inhalation or ingestion of bacilli sprayed into the atmosphere from the infected, ulcerated nasal cavities of untreated lepromatous patients. In certain parts of the world today, some communities still have a high incidence of disease—as much as 1 percent of the population. The popular belief of the high infectivity of leprosy is obviously misplaced, since in such communities more than 95 percent never develop any evidence of the disease, even though every member of the population will regularly encounter infected individuals. It is suggested that most people have complete immunity to the infection and are able to obliterate any leprosy bacilli that manage to enter the body without producing any recognizable signs and symptoms. The wide range of clinical signs of leprosy occurs in individuals whose personal immunity to infection is either incomplete or totally absent.

Patients with High but Incomplete Immunity

Patients with a less-than-perfect ability to overcome infection produce a reaction of the cell-mediated type in which epithelioid cells and Langhans' giant cells are surrounded by a mantle of lymphocytes, producing a classical tuberculoid granuloma. These patients will be dealing with very few mycobacteria. Even if the infecting load were heavy, multiplication will be prevented by the relatively high resistance; consequently, recognizable lesions will be few and almost certainly asymmetrical. Such patients will have the *pure neural* or *tuberculoid* forms of disease.

Anergic Patients (Absent Immunity)

When people are completely unable to combat infection, the organisms, entering tissues of their choice, multiply almost indefinitely. Until recently, it has been suggested that the patients had no suitable T-cells, but further knowledge of these thymus-dependent cells has shown that the T-suppressor cells are increased and the helper cells diminished in this type of individual. Whether this is immunologically important or not is immaterial to the mycobacteria, whose multiplication continues apace without provoking a tuberculoid granuloma. As time goes on, the organisms multiply to such a degree that the patient develops foreign-body granulomata in reaction to the bacillary mass, and swarms of acid-fast bacilli are enveloped by histiocytes and foam cells. Epithelioid cells and lymphocytes are conspicuous by their absence. This type of disease is called *lepromatous leprosy.*

Patients with a Small Amount of Immunity

The existence of tuberculoid and lepromatous leprosy does not mean that there is an all-or-none classification into which all infected individuals have to be confined. Many patients whose immunity is lower than that found in tuberculoid individuals but higher than that of the lepromatous will, according to their position in a spectrum ranging between these two poles, show increasing numbers of lesions and bacteria, with an intermediate type of pathology that is neither one thing or the other. In most parts of the world, these patients are said to have *borderline leprosy,* but there are still some stalwart traditionalists who prefer to say these patients have intermediate or dimorphous disease.

The Spectrum of Leprosy

Most research workers classify the disease into five basic types (see Table 6-1): the pure tuberculoid (TT) and the pure lepromatous (LL) are at opposite ends of the spectrum, while between them are various forms of borderline disease known as borderline tuberculoid (BT), borderline (BB), and borderline lepromatous (BL).

This Ridley-Jopling research classification covers almost all cases that are seen. The types of disease vary in the number of lesions present, the number of bacteria in each lesion, and the nature of the histopathology, as well as the positivity of the lepromin test (see Appendix one). A number of other diagnoses

TABLE 6-1 The Leprosy Spectrum

	Polar Tuberculoid (TT)	Borderline Tuberculoid (BT)	Borderline (BB)	Borderline Lepromatous (BL)	Polar Lepromatous (LL)	
					Multiple (nodular leproma)	or Total (diffuse lepromatosis)
Number of lesions	One or two	Few	Some	Many	Multiple (nodular leproma)	or Total (diffuse lepromatosis)
Bacterial index in untreated cases	0	1+ 2+	3+	4+	5+ (6+ occasionally seen)	
Anesthesia	Asymmetrical and early		Early occasionally seen		Symmetrical and late onset	
Pathology	Classical tuberculoid granuloma with epithelioid cells		Mixture of epithelioid and histiocytic cells		Foreign body granuloma with histiocytes and foam cells	
Lepromin test	+++ ++	+ ±	0	0	0	
Reactions	Probably never seen	Downgrading most common	Downgrading or reversal	Reversal or ENL	ENL only	ENL or Lucio phenomenon

are sometimes used (neural leprosy, indeterminate leprosy, diffuse leprosy, etc.). Their places alongside the classical spectrum will be considered later.

Clinical Features

Pure Neural Leprosy

The prediliction of *M. leprae* for nervous tissue, particularly the Schwann cell, ensures that very few cases of leprosy exist in which nerves are not demonstrably involved either clinically or histologically. Sometimes, a patient shows nerve involvement but absolutely no evidence of dermatologic lesions (Figure 6-1). Such a condition cannot occur in an anergic patient, whose inability to cope with infection would be unable to prevent skin involvement to a greater or lesser degree. A highly resistant patient, putting up a good struggle, sometimes may not be able to prevent the appearance of a single patch of tuberculoid leprosy on the skin. (Figure 6-2), and it is not surprising that occasionally this single lesion occurs in a nerve rather than in the dermis.

The disease usually affects one of the more superficial nerves, most frequently the ulnar, but also the radial, the preauricular, and the lateral poplit-

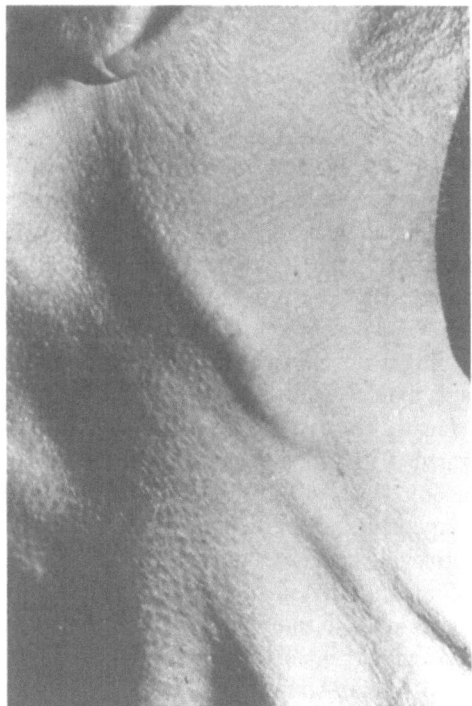

FIGURE 6-1   Neural leprosy: this patient had no lesions on his skin.

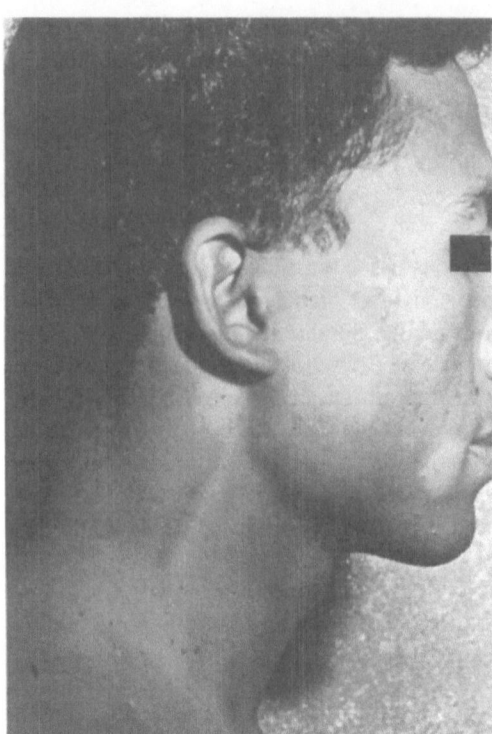

FIGURE 6-2 Neural leprosy with a single early tuberculoid lesion at the corner of the mouth.

eal. The nerve becomes thickened, harder, and sometimes more nodular than normal. Enlargement alone is totally insufficient to suggest the diagnosis, but very few nerves are both enlarged and hardened, and an enlarged, easily palpable, and nodular superficial nerve should always be suspect, especially if associated with a patch of anesthesia later followed by a gradual loss of power and ultimate wasting in a group of muscles. Skin scrapings will be negative for AFB. The lepromin test should when possible be performed—a mildly positive reaction is not unusual in residents of endemic areas, but a strongly positive test is diagnostically helpful.

Ideally, no case should be diagnosed unless a nerve biopsy has been performed. This will show a classical tuberculoid histology that, taking up a fair amount of space but confined within the fibrous perineurium, explains the enlargement and hardening of the nerve as well as the associated peripheral neurologic changes (Figure 6-4).

Similar nerve involvement associated with skin lesions can be found in tuberculoid and some types of borderline disease, producing asymmetric nerve involvement among the early clinical signs. In lepromatous patients, intraneural foreign-body granulomata slowly produce a stocking-and-glove anesthesia that extends up the limbs in association with more or less general wast-

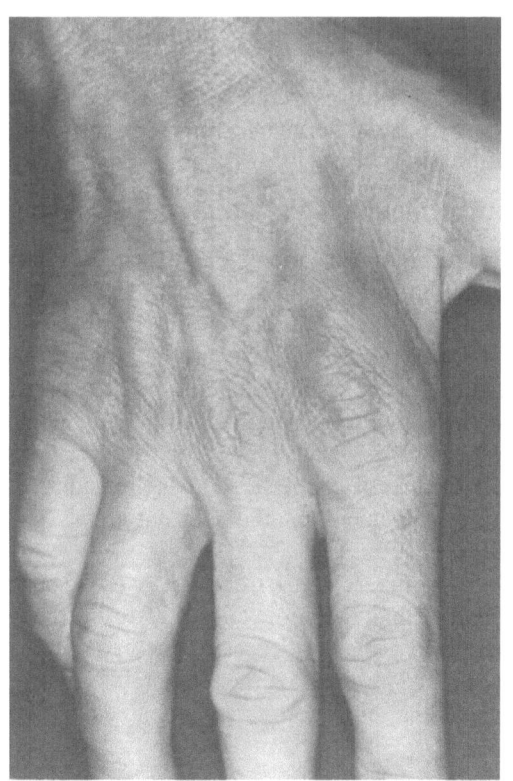

FIGURE 6-3 Neural leprosy: wasting of the interossei resulting from leprosy infection of the ulnar nerve.

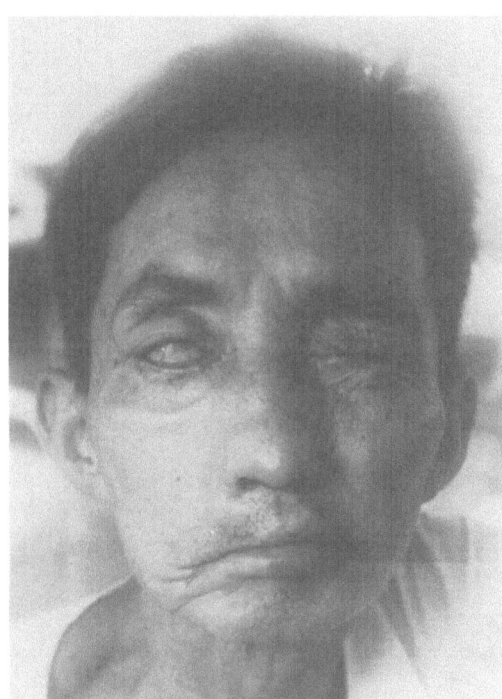

FIGURE 6-4 Facial paralysis in tuberculoid leprosy—the persistent exposure of the right cornea needs urgent attention from an ophthalmic surgeon.

ing of the muscles of the hands and feet. By the time this occurs, the patients will have had extensive lepromatous leprosy for many years.

Tuberculoid Leprosy (TT)

The polar type of tuberculoid disease is usually a rather scaly infiltrated single lesion that may be anything from 1 or 2 to 20 or 30 centimeters in diameter: such areas are invariably anesthetic. They have raised edges and, if they have attained a reasonable size, are most often found to be spreading peripherally and healing centrally. Sometimes, a few smaller lesions are present elsewhere on the body, but normally such patients do not have more than three or four plaques. Occasionally, such patches consist of small clusters of papules looking like a group of cobblestones, which histologically can be shown to have miniature tuberculoid granulomata but are too small for anesthesia to be detected (Figure 6-5).

Many tuberculoid patches are hypopigmented. If the patient is examined in direct sunlight (traditionally said to be the proper way to look at a patient suspected of having leprosy), one or two areas of hypopigmentation may be seen in the absence of other detectable change. Indeed, now and then a patient has nothing but a few hypopigmented and hypoesthetic areas.

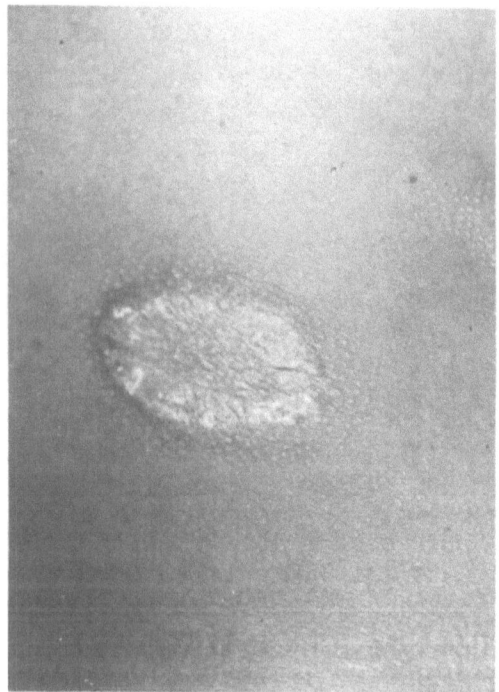

FIGURE 6-5 Tuberculoid leprosy: the patch is scaly and surrounded by cobblestone papules. A lesion consisting only of such papules is on the right.

FIGURE 6-6 Tuberculoid leprosy: the skin is slightly thickened and mildly scaly, and the
well-demarcated patch is anesthetic.

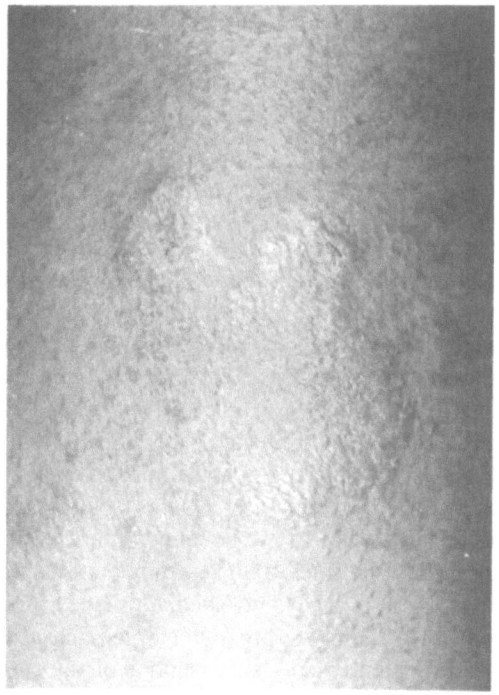

Diagnosis of tuberculoid leprosy is easy because no other skin lesion is anesthetic. When the diagnosis has been suspected, the next thing to do is to examine the patient carefully for evidence of affected nerves (Figure 6-6). An abnormal preauricular nerve may be seen crossing the sternomastoids, and by running the back of a fingernail along each clavicle, the physician may be able to detect enlargement in one or more of the fine supraclavicular nerves that course over the clavicle directly beneath the skin. The ulnar should be examined at the elbow, where it is normally palpable. If it is affected, it will not only be big and hard, but the pain that normally radiates down the limb when a normal nerve is squeezed will be diminished or absent. Enlarged superficial branches of the radial nerve can be felt crossing the end of the radius and, if one wraps one's fingers around the head of the fibula and then moves them slightly down and backwards, it is possible to detect an abnormal lateral popliteal nerve running around the neck of the fibula.

Whether or not it is possible to detect large nerves, the whole skin should be carefully examined for anesthesia. The earliest sensory change is usually a dulling of temperature appreciation, best demonstrated by asking patients to close their eyes and recognize the difference between two test-tubes, one full of crushed ice and the other of boiling water. Later loss of sensation to pin prick and cotton may be found not only in the visible patches of cutaneous disease but in other areas supplied by nerves that have not been recognized clinically as having an infection.

If more than five lesions are detected (neural or cutaneous), the patient probably does not have tuberculoid disease of the polar type.

Lepromatous Leprosy (LL)

Patients who are completely unable to combat *M. leprae* infection are of two types. A few (more common in Central America) probably have a congenital anergy and react to infection by producing a diffuse lepromatosis (see page 74), while more commonly, and much more widespread, some patients will produce a nodular lepromatous disease probably due to secondary anergy. They have a mixture of macules, papules, nodules, and diffusely infiltrated plaques scattered throughout the skin. Occasionally, particularly in the early stage, the macules are hypopigmented, but later the lesions become raised, red, and shiny, never showing any signs of epidermal involvement, such as the scaling seen in TT. They are to be found almost everywhere, but less frequently affect the palms and soles, axillae, groin, and scalp.

The face is always involved, ultimately producing a leonine facies, while the lobes of the ears are grossly enlarged and pendulous. Involvement of the forehead frequently causes destruction of the outer parts of the eyebrows (mada-

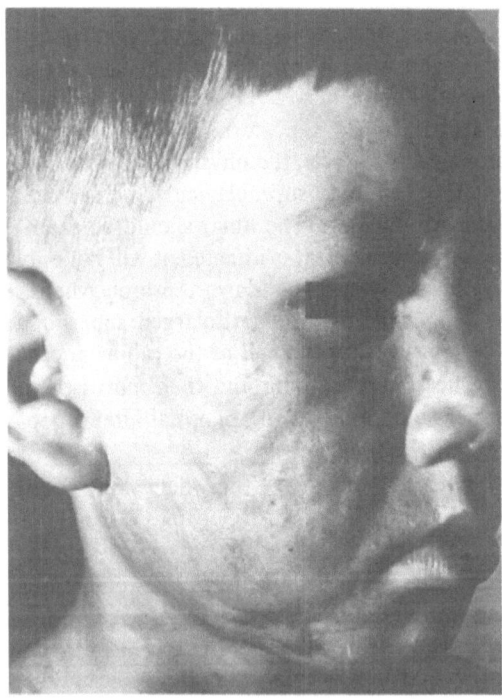

FIGURE 6-7 Early lepromatous leprosy. The earlobes and eyebrows are already involved as well as the thickening of the skin of the face. (Courtesy J. Sidney Rice, M.D. Collection of the College of Physicians of Philadelphia.)

FIGURE 6-8   Marked lepromatous leprosy affecting the lips as
well as the nose, ears, eyebrows,
and chin.

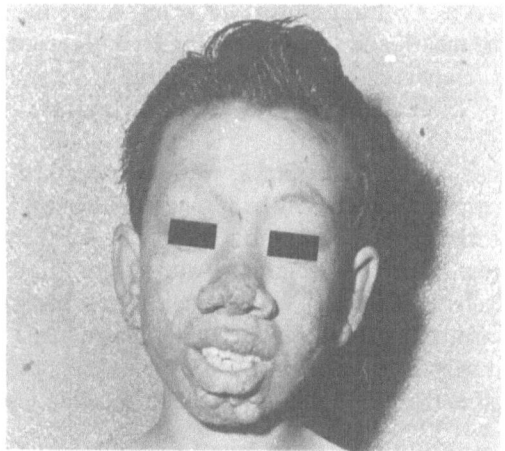

rosis), and in the later stages the whole of the eyebrow may be permanently
destroyed (Figures 6-7 to 6-9).

It is not only the skin that is affected; the nose is involved early in the course
of disease. Small ulcerated nodules produce a crusting and secretion that will
be full of AFB—some authorities believe that nasal discharge may be the

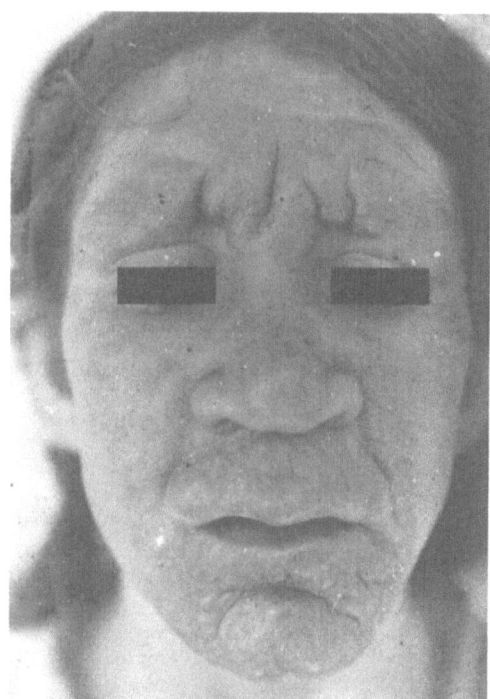

FIGURE 6-9   Leonine facies of
lepromatous leprosy.

source of all transmitted infection. Before the advent of satisfactory treatment the mouth and larynx were involved in the final stages of the disease, but this is rarely seen today.

Thickened peripheral nerves such as are seen in TT are not found in the early stages of lepromatous leprosy, unless the patient has a form of disease that has evolved from a previous borderline phase. As the disease extends, peripheral nerves slowly degenerate, starting with the hands and feet, where a stocking-and-glove anesthesia spreads up the limbs. At the same time, neuro-trophic atrophy, combined with disuse atrophy caused by muscle paralysis, leads to absorption of the small bones, particularly the phalanges. Repeated unnoticed trauma and secondary infection allow wounds of the hands and feet to penetrate deeply into the tissue, where a combination of these effects pro-duces the gross deformities that are such a feared element of the illness.

Borderline Leprosy

The different types of borderline disease are less clear than might be hoped for, as their diagnosis relies to some extent on quantity judgments.

Borderline Tuberculoid (BT)
Although they are more numerous in this group, each individual lesion is almost indistinguishable from those in TT, perhaps showing a little less scaling

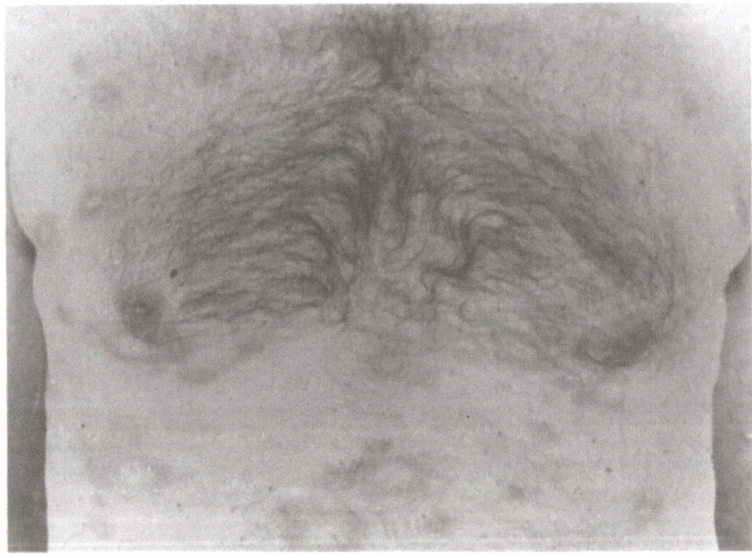

FIGURE 6-10   Borderline leprosy—note the numerous annular lesions with well-defined inner margins.

and sensory loss but still being well demarcated. If BT patients have any annular lesions (and most of them do) the outer border of the ring is clearly defined while the inner border is less clear-cut (Figure 6-10).

Lesions are asymmetrical, but hypopigmentation is less marked and erythema more frequent.

Borderline (BB)

This shows a further increase in number of lesions, of which many have a moderate degree of hypoesthesia. The patches are redder and more infiltrated than those seen in tuberculoid cases and often have annular lesions that differ from those in BT—the *outer* border will be diffuse and unclear while the *inner* border is so well marked that it has been described as having a punched-out or Swiss-cheese appearance (Figures 6-10, 6-11).

Borderline Lepromatous (BL)

This has so many nodules, papules, and plaques that at first sight it may be mistaken for LL (Figure 6-12). The lesions, however, are still somewhat asymmetrical. Madarosis, nasal ulceration, and other features of true lepromatous disease are missing. It is not unlikely that the patient will have a few annular lesions of the BB type.

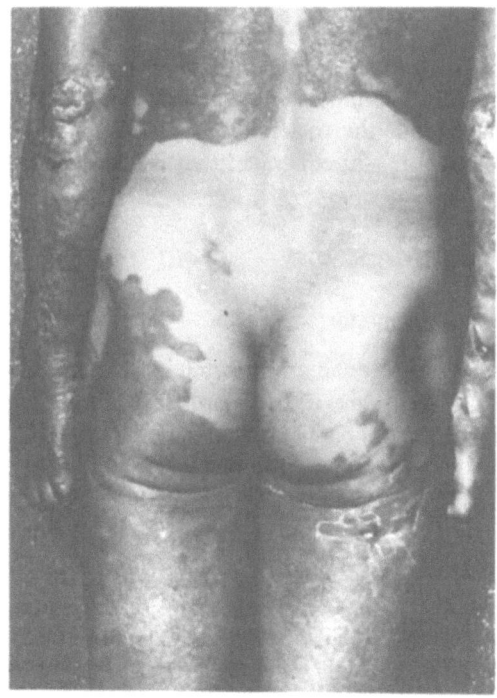

FIGURE 6-11   The clear zone in the center of a borderline lesion is sometimes called the immune zone. It is unusually extensive in this patient; elsewhere the skin has progressed to fully lepromatous disease with large nodules on the arms and deformed hands.

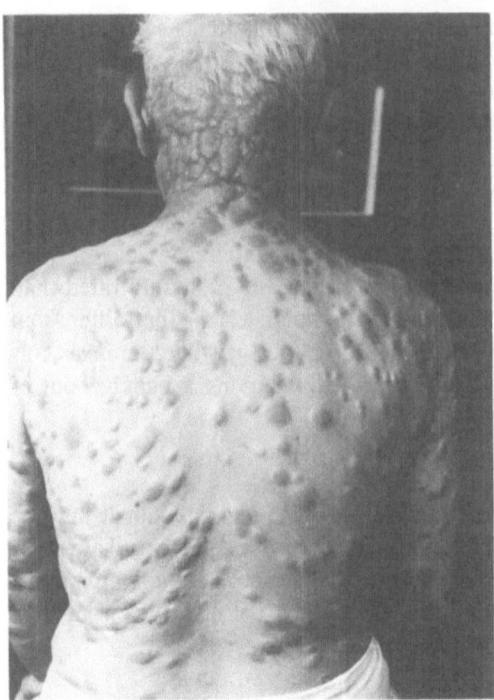

FIGURE 6-12 Borderline lepromatous disease. Multiple
nodules that have recently
become edematous and erythematous as a result of a reversal
reaction.

In all cases of borderline leprosy, the immunologic status may vary and so produce overlapping of symptoms with a neighboring type. It is often possible to combine the "colors" of the spectrum and to say that a patient has BT/BB or BL/LL—a refinement that is more elegant than necessary.

Natural History

Incubation Period

Most people who are infected by *M. leprae* never develop a recognizable disease. Even those whose insufficient immunity ensures that signs and symptoms will ultimately appear have the infection for many years before it becomes visible. The incubation period is at least five years, since it takes this long to develop in a child whose parents both have untreated lepromatous disease and who is therefore immunologically wide open to infection and lives in an area that must be profusely contaminated with the organisms. Most patients take many years longer; American soldiers who have never left the continental United States since their return from military service in the Pacific sometimes have not developed the disease for 25 years or more. It may be said that they were infected in their own country, but probability is against this.

It must be emphasized that a clinical suspicion that someone has leprosy should not be ruled out because the patient has not visited an endemic area for a long time.

Progress of Untreated Leprosy

In most parts of the world today, patients usually manage to receive some treatment; it is only in the most undeveloped areas that people are found with a history of 20 to 30 years of visible infection. Such individuals are covered with large nodules, ulceration has usually caused the nose to collapse, the palate may be perforated, the eyes destroyed, and the hands and feet mutilated beyond all recognition. LL will not get better spontaneously.

At the other pole, TT cases rarely give a history of having had the lesion for many years. Two reasons must be considered: either all cases of TT get worse and progress into borderline disease or many of these cases spontaneously resolve. The latter suggestion is more likely, and it is probable that individuals with high but incomplete immunity are sometimes able to enhance such immunity a little and overcome the disease. Doctors working in endemic areas will have seen many cases with wasting of peripheral muscles associated with an area of anesthesia and a large hardened nerve that have been present for many years. It is sometimes possible to obtain a history that a transient skin lesion was present in the past. Although TT may undergo spontaneous resolution, this possibility should never be invoked as an excuse to withold treatment in case the patient's history is unreliable and the disease is continuing.

Clinical progress of borderline leprosy may follow a much more variable course. Sometimes the patient's disease remains more or less stable for many years, but as the immunity is less fixed than that seen in polar disease abrupt changes in the clinical and histologic picture are by no means unknown. These are usually referred to as lepra reactions.

Reactions in Leprosy

Most skin diseases either get worse steadily, get better steadily, or remain unchanged. Borderline leprosy does not necessarily follow any of these examples. For a long time, it has been known that there may be a sudden severe exacerbation of the preexisting leprosy lesions. This sometimes occurs before treatment has been initiated (stimulating an urgent search for medical assistance), but may also be seen in patients who are receiving effective antileprosy therapy. It has taken a long time for leprologists to realize that although such incidents look the same, two different reactions are involved: one associated with a diminution of the previously existing immunity and the other accompanying an enhancement of immunity. It goes without saying that these two reactions cannot occur together.

Downgrading

Patients who have never sought medical advice for their leprosy are often stimulated to do so by the sudden explosive exacerbation of all the lesions on the skin, which, whether they are few or many, suddenly become much redder and more swollen than they have ever been before. The dermatologic aggravation will be associated with severe nerve pain if a similar edematous reaction occurs in an intra-neural lesion; foot-drop, wrist-drop, or facial palsy can develop rapidly, and even urgent treatment may not prevent permanent paralysis (Figure 6-4). This used to be called the downgrading reaction, but the use of the word *reaction* is not logical since what has happened is that the patient's immunity has undergone a sudden collapse and progress toward lepromatous disease has been speeded up. Downgrading cannot occur if a patient is receiving effective antibacterial treatment.

Reversal Reaction

Unfortunately, the exacerbation seen in a downgrading patient is not unique. Patients whose immunity suddenly improves will experience a clinically similar and equally rapid swelling and erythema of all their preexisting lesions. Occasionally, this stretches the skin to such a degree that the epidermis ruptures, and ulceration occurs.

If this happens in a leprosarium, where patients are regularly biopsied on admission, it will be found that such cases starting with a pathology of BB or BL have developed a pathology much closer to the tuberculoid pole (when the reaction has subsided). This reversal reaction is associated with a much more rapid reduction in bacterial number than may be expected under the normal course of therapy.

Most often reversal reactions occur some three to six months after the start of effective treatment, probably because treatment has reduced the viable bacterial load to such an extent that the T-cells have been able to work more effectively.

Progress in Treated Cases

When suitable antileprosy therapy is administered to a new case, the lesions will slowly resolve and the dermatologic changes will begin to disappear. In tuberculoid patients, usually nothing is visible after three years, and most lepromatous patients will be considerably improved after seven years, the infiltrating granulomata having dissolved. Unfortunately, the existence for so long of tumors stretching and destroying dermal connective tissue often means that lepromatous patients are left with a lax, wrinkled skin on the face and softly pendulous earlobes, as well as the missing eyebrows that are such a common feature of the disease.

Neurologic lesions usually do not improve. Sometimes patches of anesthesia diminish in area, probably because of reinervation from unaffected nerves spreading in from the periphery, and small lesions 1 to 2 cm in diameter may regain sensation entirely.

Muscle wasting is unaltered, and the sad fact remains that neurotrophic changes of the hands, penetrating infection, and repeated ulceration of the feet cause the orthopedic aspects of leprosy to progress unchanged.

Recurrent attacks of infection of the feet are often associated with lymphangitis, which may ultimately obliterate the lymphatics, and in an unfortunate few cause the unpleasant and irremediable complication known as lymphostasis verrucosa or mossy foot (Figures 6-13, 6-14).

Erythema Nodosum Leprosum

Perhaps the most serious complication of all and certainly the one that is most liable to have a fatal outcome is the condition known as erythema nodosum leprosum (ENL), which was originally described by Murata in Japan in 1912. It is limited to LL and BL cases and has, along with other reactions, been the subject of a tremendous amount of confused thinking.

In the section on bacteriology (see page 67) it will be explained in greater detail that microscopic studies of AFB obtained by skin smear will show two sorts of organisms, those that take suitable stains in a smooth, uniform way (called solid-staining mycobacteria and known to be viable) and others whose

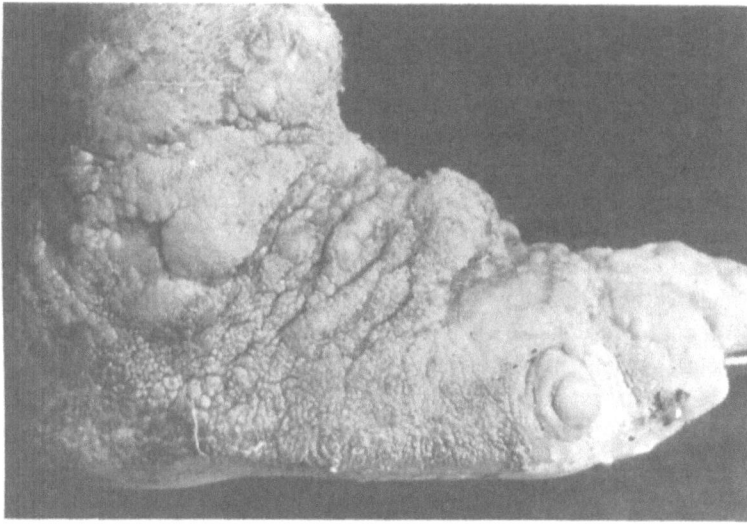

FIGURE 6-13   Mossy foot (lymphostasis verrucosa) in a patient with long-standing lepromatous leprosy and extensive anesthesia.

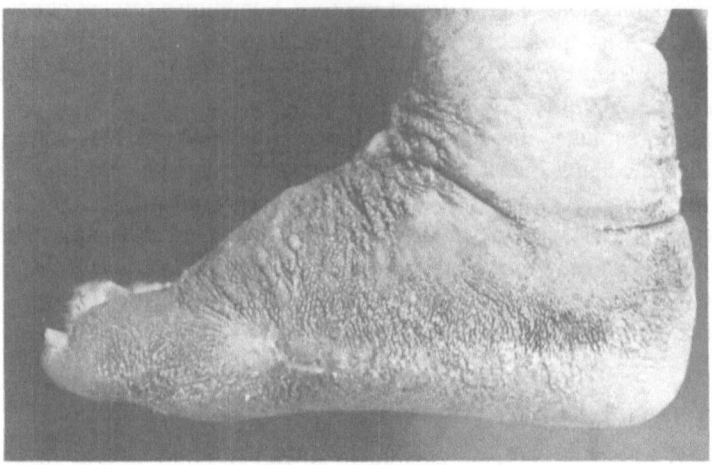

FIGURE 6-14   Another example of the mossy foot.

cytoplasm looks beaded and broken, which are known as fragmented organisms, are nonviable, and are in the process of disintegration. Untreated patients have a fairly high percentage of viable organisms, called the morphologic index (MI). Within a few months of the start of satisfactory therapy all organisms become fragmented: the morphologic index falls to zero. ENL begins at this time.

For reasons that are difficult to explain, dead leprosy bacilli take a very long time to disintegrate, and the slow release of bacterial toxins from these disintegrating organisms sets up a form of allergic vasculitis that may vary from mild to exceedingly severe. Some leprologists have claimed the ENL is caused by dapsone and have even urged that sulfone therapy be stopped. This is completely illogical, since dapsone given for other diseases in equal or higher dosage for a similar or longer period does not produce ENL. The drug is nonetheless implicated, however, because without its therapeutic effect *M. leprae* would not have been killed and the subsequent release of high quantities of bacterial toxin would not have occurred. In the last few years it has been shown that people with lepromatous disease develop ENL when treated with other successful antileprosy medications. Patients who get this complication must be clearly told that it is no more than an unfortunate reaction to the effective killing of the acid-fast bacilli.

As the name suggests, the basic lesion is a small red papule that is usually painful. In contrast to downgrading and reversal reactions, these lesions do not involve the ordinary leprosy nodule but may be seen anywhere on the skin, including the face. It has become an unfortunate habit of some workers to refer to this condition as erythema nodosum. Such a practice is to be condemned, as erythema nodosum is a well-known dermatologic condition of different etiology that affects different areas (common on the shin and never on the face) and has a different, purplish, color.

ENL starts some 6 to 12 months after the start of treatment—about half of all LL cases get it during the course of treatment and about 20 percent of BL cases are affected.

It starts modestly with a few small, painful nodules not much more than a centimeter in diameter. Sometimes, with the help of a little therapy, this is all that happens. Often it becomes more severe. Increasing numbers of lesions are associated with mildly raised temperature, and later there may be a persistant, high, swinging fever and recurrent eruption of nodules, each individual lesion lasting from 10 to 14 days. In the most severe type the nodules will ulcerate, discharging a mucopurulent necrotic material and finishing with a ragged irregular scar. This is fortunately rare.

Not only is the skin involved: superficial lymph nodes and peripheral nerves may become enlarged and painful, and enlargement of the spleen and liver, swelling of the testes, ascites, and pleural effusion may all be associated with a fever that can continue for years. Finally, the bacterial index becomes negative, and at this time, there being no more bacterial toxins available to cause trouble, the ENL will subside. This persistant disease may lead to secondary amyloidosis, which in the 1920s and 1930s was a common cause of death from leprosy.

Differential Diagnosis

The multiplicity of signs and symptoms produced by *M. leprae* means that in various patients widely differing disease may cause diagnostic confusion.

Pure Neural Leprosy

An enlarged and hardened nerve is very unusual. The condition known as familial hypertrophic interstitial neuritis (Déjérine's disease) will show thickening of peripheral nerves with sensory loss and motor change, but the nerves themselves are not particularly hard, and usually several are involved at the same time. This will not be the case in pure neural leprosy, while in tuberculoid disease, if several nerves are affected, there will also be diagnostic skin signs.

Trauma may damage a nerve but not cause it to be enlarged. Syringomyelia, familial radicular neuropathy, and primary amyloidosis of peripheral nerves have all at times caused diagnostic confusion.

Tuberculoid Leprosy

An established patch of tuberculoid leprosy should never be mistaken for anything else; whether it is scaly (usual) or smooth (rare), it is invariable anesthetic and so unlike any other dermatosis. It is, of course, necessary to test the apparently normal skin on the same limb as well as the visible lesion to ensure that anesthesia is not generalized but limited to the patch.

Despite the histologic similarities between tuberculoid leprosy, lupus vulgaris, and lupoid leishmaniasis, clinical confusion is unlikely to occur, since most tuberculoid granulomata show apple-jelly nodules in an extending scar, a presentation that is never seen in leprosy.

Borderline Disease

All forms of borderline disease may be missed by doctors who, having suspected that the patient had leprosy, rule out the possibility because the lesions are not anesthetic. It must always be remembered that many types of leprosy are not anesthetic.

Annular lesions of BT and BB can be confused with annular psoriasis or a centripetal tinea corporis. In both these conditions, the epidermis is demonstrably involved. In borderline disease, there is no epidermal change.

Late yaws and certain forms of leishmaniasis may present difficult diagnostic problems. In areas where two of these diseases exist simultaneously, skin scraping and biopsy may be needed to clarify matters.

Lepromatous Disease

Anergic leishmaniasis, post-kala-azar dermal leishmaniasis, late yaws, and various lymphomas, including mycosis fungoides, may all be confused with lepromatous leprosy, but nodular sarcoidosis is rarely extensive enough to be a problem. In all these cases, nasal ulceration, madarosis, contractures, and neural changes will help to confirm the diagnosis.

Downgrading and Reversal Reactions
These frequently occur in patients already diagnosed, in which case problems should not arise, but if a patient is seen for the first time while in reaction, sarcoidosis or lymphoma may be suspected. A careful history will reveal the existence of skin lesions prior to the exacerbation and lead to a careful search for neurologic signs.

Erythema Nodosum Leprosum
ENL is nothing like erythema nodosum and only occurs in patients with extensive lepromatous disease. Diagnosis should never be in doubt if the patient has nodular disease, but may be missed if it is associated with diffuse lepromatosis. Patients with transient painful nodules and a persistent fever may be suspected to have a severe vasculitis or even polyarteritis nodosa, but diffuse thickening of the earlobes and madarosis will usually be present. Routine bacterial and pathologic studies will confirm the presence of diffuse lepromatosis.

Investigations

Bacteriology

In most bacterial diseases, an unsuccessful search for the causative organism will raise doubts as to the accuracy of the diagnosis. This is not necessarily true in leprosy; not only is it impossible to find any organism in many tuberculoid cases, but even in those patients with a profusion of organisms, in vitro culture is invariably negative.

A search for *M. leprae* must be carried out to confirm that the clinical classification of the patient has been as accurate as possible. Tissue smears should always be taken by the skin-slit technique (see Appendix one). If only a few lesions are present smears should be taken from them all. In lepromatous individuals six smears should be taken: from the left earlobe, the right earlobe, the left elbow, the back, the right arm, and one of the legs. In most cases, lesions should be tested, but it is wise to take one of the smears from apparently normal skin, as the presence of bacilli in such skin will indicate that the patient has LL rather than BL.

Unfortunately, this test is not particularly scientific, since an unmeasured quantity of tissue fluid is spread over an unmeasured area on the glass slide and the number of AFB in each smear will depend not only on the lesion but also on the technician. It is recommended that the organisms be counted and reported on Ridley's logarithmic index (see appendix one), in which the bacterial index (BI—total bacterial number in each smear) is graded as 1+ if a single organism is detected in 100 oil-immersion fields and 5+ if more than 100 bacilli are seen in each field. The use of the logarithmic scale means that when the BI falls from 5+ to 4+ there has been a 90 percent reduction in organisms. If the average BI of six smears is taken, a fairly reliable graph can be drawn of the patient's progress, particularly if the same technique is always used. In this way, satisfactory coordination will be found with diagnostic classification. TT patients will show completely negative smears, and the BI will rise (as is shown in Table 6-1) to an average of 5+ in cases of untreated LL.

Unfortunately, the presence of bacilli is not an indication of the activity of the disease. *M. leprae* has a cell wall that is much less fragile than that found in other organisms, and instead of disappearing rapidly as happens after treatment with gonorrhea or tuberculosis, the dead organisms disintegrate with such painful slowness that it may take up to ten years for a heavily infected lepromatous patient to become smear negative despite the continuous use of a completely successful therapy. Fortunately, however, there is another way to assess progress.

Even when Dr. Hansen first saw the bacilli in 1873, he noticed that some had a beaded appearance and suggested that they might be dead. In the past 30 years, it has been recognized that, when a skin smear is stained and suitably decolorized, some of the organisms stain uniformly while others do not. Solid-staining bacilli, injected into the footpad of a thymectomized and irradiated mouse, will multiply, but fragmented organisms will not. It is believed that the solid-staining bacilli are viable and the fragmented ones are not.

A new method of counting the organisms has therefore been devised that has the advantage of being more informative. In each smear, 100 consecutive, clearly visible organisms are examined, and the number of those staining solidly is recorded. The morphologic index (MI) is the percentage of viable bacilli present in a smear. If six smears are studied, both the BI and the MI should be recorded for each site. This must be done at the start of treatment, after six weeks, three months, six months, and then at yearly intervals. An untreated patient will have some 20 to 40 percent solid organisms (even mycobacteria are not immortal), and with satisfactory therapy the MI will fall to zero within six months. Slowly the BI will follow suit, and Ridley's logarithmic index will be recognizably lower after a year's therapy.

It is now possible to grow *M. leprae* not only in the footpads of mice but in armadilloes and other animals. The expense of such techniques, however, makes them unsuitable for any but research purposes.

Histopathology

It should not be necessary to biopsy a tuberculoid lesion; anesthesia of the plaque is total confirmation of the diagnosis. In other types of disease, the histopathology will be helpful.

In the tuberculoid cases a classical tuberculoid histology (epithelioid cells, Langhans' cells, and lymphocytes) will be found in the dermis and may also be detected in any peripheral nerve seen in the section. Caseation, which may occur in neural leprosy, is very rare indeed in the skin, and if seen is much more suggestive of tuberculosis. Tuberculosis, however, will never affect a nerve.

As the degree of immunity diminishes, epithelioid cells give way, and the presence of histiocytes, foreign-body giant cells, foam cells containing large clusters of mycobacteria known as globi, and an almost total disappearance of lymphocytes will produce a diagnostic pathology.

In downgrading and reversal reactions, leprosy can still be recognized, but there is in addition vascular dilation and edema running parallel with the erythematous swelling of the clinical lesions. At the same time, the change in clinical immunity that has been responsible for such exacerbations will cause an unexpected increase or decrease in bacilli and also a change in the type of granuloma.

Erythema nodosum leprosum may be seen fortuitously in a routine lepromatous section. Larger lesions that have been specifically biopsied show the same changes only more marked. Numerous polymorphonuclear leukocytes will be present predominantly in the early stages, and later a vasculitis is seen in some of the superficial blood vessels, which also show bacterial infiltration in their walls. In the most severe cases, necrotizing lesions may develop in the dermis, associated with subsequent epidermal necrosis.

Lepromin Test

This should be of assistance in confirming the diagnosis; unfortunately, sometimes tuberculoid patients have a false negative reaction, and while false positives are rare in lepromatous cases, a contaminated needle may produce an infected papule that can be misread as positive and cause some diagnostic perturbation.

If lepromin is not easily available, its absence need not be mourned.

Treatment

The treatment of leprosy will always take a long time. Because the clinical appearance only slowly improves, it may take many months before a physician can decide clinically whether there has been any improvement. Evidence of successful therapy must therefore depend on laboratory investigations.

Dapsone

For many years, diamino-diphenylsulfone was the only successful drug and one that was apparently invariably effective. In the 1960s and 1970s, many dosages were advocated, but it is now generally agreed that all cases of leprosy should be given 100 mg dapsone daily and that this dose should neither be increased or decreased without overriding reason. To follow the patient's progress the BI and the MI should be taken regularly. The morphologic index usually falls to zero within six months; in the past few years, however, it has shown that some leprosy bacilli are sulfone resistant.

The first cases of this type were found in patients in whom, despite prolonged therapy, organisms had been able to flourish and whose MI was 20 to 30 percent. Such cases showed hard, shiny nodules, usually darker and less erythematous than ordinary lepromatous lesions, with an overgrowth of fibroblastic histiocytes complicating the histology (Figures 6-15, 6-16). More recently, it has been found that in some people sulfone resistance is present *ab initio;* the disease persists and the MI remains unchanged despite what is believed to be suitable sulfone therapy. In these cases, the footpad technique demonstrates that mice receiving sulfone in their diet are unable to combat the AFB infection.

Before the recognition of sulfone resistance, the search for other antileprosy drugs was somewhat desultory, because they were only needed if the patient was sulfone sensitive (a rare occurrence). More recently, it has become urgently necessary to find other successful medications.

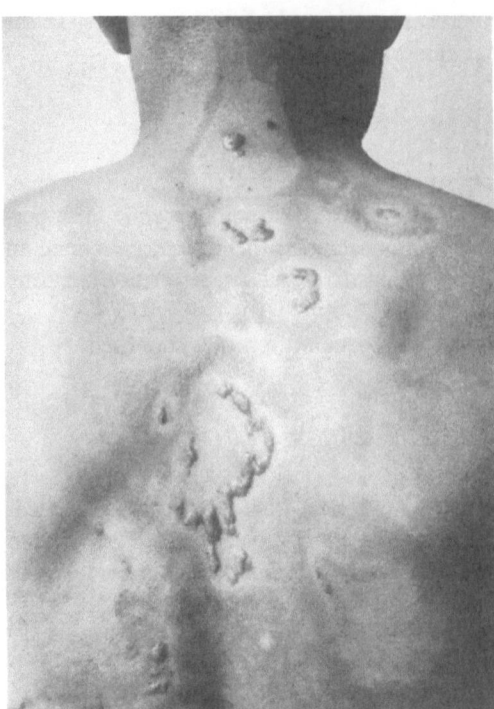

FIGURE 6-15 Sulfone-resistant leprosy with hard, dark, and shiny nodules, returning in the hypochromic sites of previous infection.

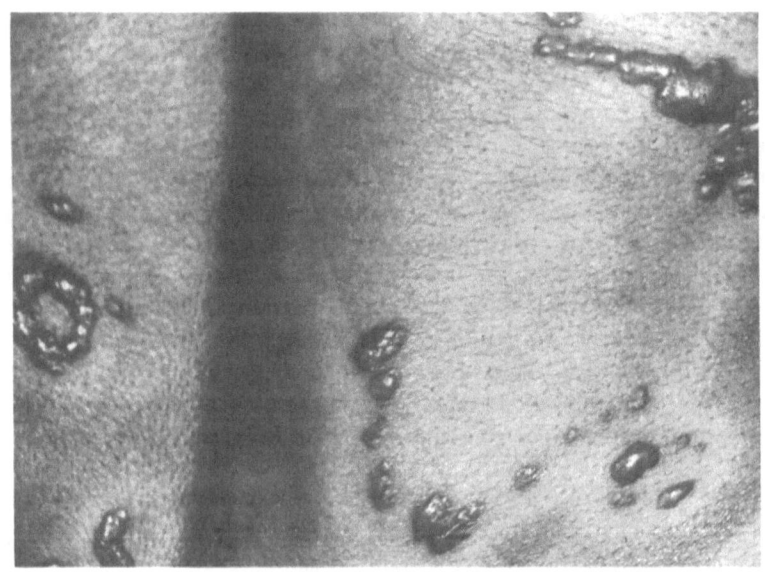

FIGURE 6-16   Close-up of sulfone-resistant nodules (see Figure 6-15).

Clofazimine

A riminophenazine dye, clofazimine is equally successful in causing a reduction of the MI to zero within three to four months. Because this dye stains the skin red and the leprosy lesions a slate grey color, however, it is less than wholeheartedly accepted by Caucasians, Chinese, Koreans, and Japanese; Africans and southern Indians usually find the treatment acceptable. One hundred milligrams given three times a day indefinitely will be as successful as sulfone, but some unpleasant side effects (particularly necrosis of abdominal lymph nodes) make it necessary to reduce treatment to 100 mg daily if it is used for more than three months.

Rifampin

This expensive drug, when given in doses of 600 mg daily, produces a fall in the MI to zero in less than six weeks (faster than any other therapy), but if it is continued for a long time, side effects (nausea, abdominal pain, and even toxic changes in the liver and kidney) are not infrequent.

Bacterial Resistance

Sporadic reports of bacterial resistance both to clofazimine and to rifampin make monotherapy no longer to be relied on. Because the newer medications are very expensive, however, the less affluent countries may well be unable to afford to use effective polytherapy.

Routine Treatment

The following routine is suggested for lepromatous disease: rifampin 1,800 mg to be given once a month for a year in addition to the standard dapsone 100 mg daily and clofazimine 100 mg three times a day to be used for three months. If this polytherapy is successful and the MI falls to zero it may well be possible after the first year of treatment to maintain the patients on dapsone alone, provided that a careful three-month check on the MI shows no evidence of increasing numbers of *M. leprae*.

In paucibacillary cases of leprosy (TT-BB), treatment with sulfone alone will be satisfactory.

Reversal and Downgrading

These exacerbations if limited to the skin would not be particularly important, but when such reactions occur in a nerve urgent treatment is needed to reduce the intraneural edema as quickly as possible and so present permanent nerve paralysis. Corticosteroids must be used, as well as prednisone 50 mg daily for a week, reduced to 40 mg for a further week and then 20 mg indefinitely until the reaction has subsided. This is best given by injection, but the dose is the same for oral or systemic therapy.

Under no circumstances should antileprosy therapy be hindered.

Erythema Nodosum Leprosum

This is the unfortunate side effect of a necessary process (the elimination of *M. leprae*), and antileprosy treatment must not be interrupted.

In early, mild cases of ENL chloroquine tablets two or three times a day have been used to relieve the condition, and the injection of stibophen (fouadine) 1 to 3 ml on alternate days may also be of help.

More severe cases needed, until recently, corticosteroid therapy, often for many years. These gravely ill patients with recurrent attacks of high fever were given prednisone, usually not much more than 20 mg daily, in the hope that steroid side effects would be less serious than the amyloidosis that develops in long-standing untreated cases.

Pain and swelling of peripheral nerves due to ENL inside the nerve used to be treated with intraneural injections of hydrocortisone combined with hyaluronidase, but this exquisitely painful treatment is no longer necessary.

Thalidomide

The recognition by Jacob Sheskin that thalidomide is useful in ENL was of major importance. In 1964, when given as a sedative to patients with severe ENL, it was found to have a dramatic effect on the reaction. Worldwide experience has now confirmed that doses ranging from 100 to 500 mg, according to the severity of the ENL, will completely suppress the signs and symptoms. It has to be given for a long time, but provided that suitable precautions are taken in women to ensure that pregnancy is avoided, it is undoubtedly true that thalidomide is at present the drug of choice for ENL.

It has no effect on the progress of leprosy itself or on downgrading and reversal reactions, and, somewhat surprisingly, it is of no therapeutic help for other forms of allergic vasculitis.

Thalidomide is not always easy to obtain, so the address of the manufacturers is included in Appendix two.

Orthopedic and Plastic Surgery

The deformities produced by leprosy need surgical assistance. Replacement of eyebrows, repair of ectropion, reduction of enlarged earlobes, correction of interosseal wasting, and tendon transplants for wrist-drop or foot-drop all challenge the inventiveness of orthopedic and plastic surgeons, whose enthusiasm sometimes persuades them to embark on operative procedures while the disease is still active. It is wiser to wait until one can be sure that the disease will not continue to progress after surgery.

Follow-up

It is always necessary to follow up leprosy cases with more than usual care. Patients should be taught to view any exacerbation of their dermatosis as being potentially serious and to seek advice at the earliest possible moment. It is not unknown for individuals to go into a reversal reaction and develop permanent nerve palsy without referring to their medical adviser.

In the later progress of lepromatous patients, after the lesions have more or less subsided, an eruption of hard, shiny nodules may mean that sulfone resistance is developing. The MI must be taken from these nodules, as in the early stages resistance is not widespread and other areas may not yet be involved.

Duration of Treatment

Not all cases need to be treated for the same length of time. Tuberculoid patients rarely need to continue treatment for more than two years after the total disappearance of skin lesions. Further medication will not modify the neuromuscular changes.

Borderline cases will take longer to resolve; it is wise to treat them for two to three more years. Lepromatous patients should be treated for life, not because the disease is incurable, but because patients with lepromatous disease do not acquire immunity and it is by no means impossible for them to get leprosy again. This will be particularly true for those who live in leprosaria.

During follow-up, a few nodules of ENL may continue to appear. This should not be surprising, as even six negative skin smears are not a complete reflection of the bacillary status of the whole patient, and scattered bacilli that are disintegrating more slowly than their colleagues may stimulate a few lesions of ENL after the patient is apparently cured.

Some Leprosy Variants

Indeterminate Leprosy

Many cases of leprosy start with areas of hypopigmentation that in the earliest stages are not anesthetic. As such lesions are frequently on the face they are usually not biopsied, but if a section is taken AFB may not be seen and the pathology may simply show a nonspecific lymphocytic inflammation. Many doctors call such lesions indeterminate leprosy, but in various parts of the world leprologists seem to use the term for different things. In Africa thousands of cases diagnosed as indeterminate leprosy are said to clear up spontaneously while in India other workers claim that only 50% of such cases get better after several years of treatment.

It is urged that the diagnosis of leprosy be made only when there is incontrovertible evidence: if it is only *suspected* that an individual will later develop the disease, diagnosis and treatment should be withheld until confirmatory evidence is forthcoming. All patients with bacterial or pathologic evidence of leprosy should of course be properly treated, but hypopigmentation and scaliness alone are *not* sufficient bases for the diagnosis of any sort of leprosy. It is suspected that at various times pityriasis alba, vitiligo, and other hypopigmented dermatoses have been misdiagnosed. We would prefer the term indeterminate leprosy to fall into abeyance. Patients proved to have leprosy should be suitably classified, and in all other cases the diagnosis of leprosy should not be invoked.

Diffuse Lepromatosis

In 1852, Lucio in Mexico described a special form of lepromatous leprosy that showed a diffuse general infiltration of the skin without formation of nodules or tubercles at any time during its evolution. The disease is obviously the result of a primary and total anergy of the patient and is exceedingly rare outside Mexico and Central America. It is usually associated with marked madarosis and destruction of the nasal septum. In young men the beard often fails to develop. In older patients diffuse infiltration may smooth out the age-lines on the face, producing an unexpectedly youthful appearance, sometimes called *lepra bonita*—the pretty leprosy.

The annals of leprosy are studded with reports of these patients, whose disease remains undiagnosed for years; by the time it is recognized the patient usually has a generalized sensory anesthesia most noticeable on the arms and legs.

The Lucio Phenomenon

Another remarkable feature of this strange variant of lepromatous leprosy is a complication that has become less common since the advent of sulfone. Usually called the Lucio phenomenon or erythema necrotisans, it is unique to diffuse lepromatosis. Starting with small outbreaks, acute eruptions become more and more numerous, particularly on the forearms and legs. They are variable and bizarre in shape, often irregular or even triangular. Starting with a well-defined pinkish, painful patch that is not usually infiltrated, a few days later a darker area appears in the center of the lesion, soon forming a small, dry scab that later drops off to leave an insignificant scar. Larger lessions may be bullous, which on bursting leave ulceration with a jagged edge surrounded by an inflammatory zone. Before the advent of sulfone it was said that death occurred within six months of the outbreak of such ulcerating lesions, which histologically resemble a severe form of erythema multiforme produced by necrotising lesions in blood vessels whose walls are packed with *M. leprae*. Secondary infection, pyoderma, and amyloidosis follow rapidly.

The differential diagnosis between this and ENL is easy, as the Lucio phenomenon only occurs as a late complication of untreated diffuse lepromatosis while ENL follows the initiation of successful therapy. If diffuse lepromatosis were regularly diagnosed early in its course, the Lucio phenomen would be prevented by effective antileprosy treatment. As it is, the outbreak of these sores and ulcers causes the patient to seek medical assistance. Sometimes antileprosy therapy has to be supplemented with corticosteroids, but it seems that thalidomide is not helpful.

Ulceration of the Skin

The skin of leprosy patients has many opportunities to ulcerate: it may break down in severe reversal reaction or downgrading; ENL can sometimes be necrotic, and the Lucio phenomen almost always ulcerates, healing with ragged white scars.

Ulceration of the feet may be associated with diffuse or localized nerve involvement. A dropped foot usually follows downgrading or reversal in a lateral popliteal nerve; contracture of the originally paralyzed muscles will lead to neurotrophic ulceration on the part of the deformed foot that is most damaged when walking. The symmetrical anesthesia in lepromatous illness ensures that the patient does not know that the sole has been damaged. As a result, infection is not associated with normal pain and discomfort, but penetrates deeply to give swelling of the foot and a plantar ulcer. Probing the lesion will reveal sinuses leading down to necrotic bony fragments. Such ulcers will never heal unless widespread curettage of the sinuses and removal of all the necrotic tissue is followed by immobilization of the foot until fibrosis has replaced necrosis. In such cases, orthopedic surgeons and physiotherapists can combine to produce suitable footwear that, by extending the weight-bearing area of the foot, will reduce the chance of further ulceration.

Leprosy Alopecia

It is often said that leprosy does not cause hair loss, but there are two exceptions to this rule. In diffuse lepromatosis, the scalp, too, is involved—up to 20% of such patients in Mexico show a diffuse thinning of the scalp hair, especially over the occiput and nape of the neck.

Many years ago, Mitsuda described an alopecia in Japanese with severe lepromatous leprosy (not the diffuse type) in which most of the hair falls out, leaving on each side of the scalp a treelike pattern where the hair grows immediately over the temporal arteries and their branches.

All the usual forms of alopecia may occur in leprosy patients, but these have no particular etiologic connection.

Ichthyosis

In all forms of leprosy anesthesia the subsequent reduction of perspiration may not be noticed by patients, but they often complain of increased dryness of the skin. Patients who originally had ichthyosis will find the condition to be more

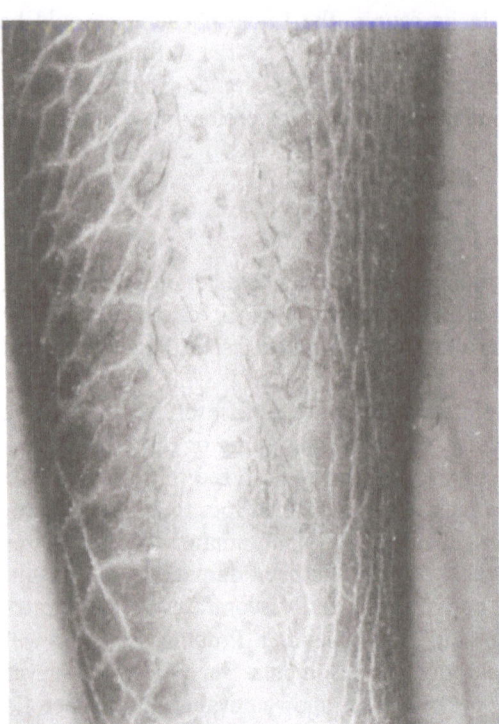

FIGURE 6-17 Ichthyosis of the shin secondary to lepromatous leprosy and aggravated by clofazimine therapy.

severe than before, while often in lepromatous patients, a severe secondary ichthyosis develops on the legs. (Figure 6-17). It has been suggested that clofazimine also causes ichthyosis, but probably the discoloration of the skin simply makes already established scaliness more visible.

Patients will have to soak the affected areas in water to rehydrate the keratin layer and then apply some form of emollient to reduce evaporation. Ten percent urea creams are sometimes useful, and bath oils will also be helpful.

Selected Readings

Barnhill, RL, McDougall, AC: Thalidomide—use and possible mode of action in reactional lepromatous leprosy. *J Am Acad Dermatol* 1982; 7:317.

Frenken, JH: *Diffuse Leprosy of Lucio and Latapi.* Orangestaad, Aruba, DeWit Inc., 1963.

Harboe, M: Significance of antibody studies in leprosy and experimental models of the disease. *Int J Leprol* 1982; 50:342.

Jopling, WH, Morgan-Hughes, JP: Pure neural tuberculoid leprosy. *Br Med J* 1965; 2:799.

Kundo, KK, Ghosh, D: Observations on clinical manifestations of primary polyneuritic types of leprosy. *Indian J Dermatol Venereol* 1970; 15:45.

Moller-Christensen, V: *Bone Changes in Leprosy*. Copenhagen, Munksgaard, 1961.

Pettit, JHS, Rees, RJW, Ridley, DS: Studies on sulfone resistant leprosy. I—detection of cases. *Int J Leprol* 1966; 29:375.

Pettit, JHS, Waters, MFR: The etiology of erythema nodosum leprosum. *Int J Leprol* 1967; 35:1.

Rea, TH, Ridley, DS: Lucio's phenomenon: A comparative histological study. *Int J Leprol* 1979; 47:161.

Ridley, DS, Jopling, WH: A classification of leprosy for research purposes. *Int J Leprol* 1960; 28:254.

Sheskin, J: Thalidomide in the treatment of lepra reaction. *Clin Pharmacol Therapeut* 1965; 6:303.

Skinsnes, OK: Epidemiology and decline of leprosy in Asia. *Int J Dermatol* 1983; 22:348

CHAPTER 7

Buruli Ulcer
(Mycobacterium Ulcerans)

For many years, this easily recognizable ulcer has had no commonly accepted dermatologic name. Recently, the tendency to call it Buruli ulcer has become more widespread, and under this name the condition will be discussed.

Originally recognized in Australia, it was further studied in Uganda (from an area near Buruli along the Victoria Nile). Since that time cases have been seen in Papua, New Guinea, Malaysia, Mexico, most of central Africa including Nigeria, and the northern parts of South America, including French Guiana. It is believed that with wider recognition of the condition, other foci will be found in countries in which the tropical equatorial forest is a feature of the landscape. Probably no case will occur that is actually acquired in temperate or colder zones.

This does not mean that the ulcers cannot be seen in unexpected places; at least one worker in the United States Peace Corps has taken his ulcer back to the United States, and a Buruli ulcer has also been recognized in France in a patient who had worked in the Congo.

Etiology

A mycobacterium, later named *Mycobacterium ulcerans,* was originally detected in association with skin ulceration in a patient living in the vicinity of Bairnsdale in Victoria, Australia (sometimes the organism is referred to as the Bairnsdale bacillus.) It is an acid-alcohol-fast organism, ranging from 1 to 4 μ long and 0.4 μ in diameter, and is strongly Gram positive (thus differentiating it from *M. leprae* or *M. tuberculosis.*) While at 37°C, inocula may occasionally produce a sparse growth after 12 weeks' incubation, it grows best at 32°C taking 3 to 4 weeks on Lowenstein-Jensen medium to produce a buff-colored, hard, flaky colony. If the organism is injected into the footpad of a mouse,

within 3 weeks swelling and ulceration will develop. If it is injected intraperi-
toneally into a mouse, gross generalized edema develops in the subcutaneous
tissue with exudates into the pleural and peritoneal cavities. Both these phenomena are believed to be unique to *M. ulcerans.*

There is no certain evidence as to the method of transmission of the disease.
It is usually seen in the swampy neighborhood of a sluggish, winding river, and,
as the inhabitants of infected communities are usually sparsely clothed,
patients sometimes suggest that bites (mosquitoes, red ants, or even cock-
roaches) may spread the disease, while cuts from plants and grasses have also
been blamed. As most ulcers occur on the knee, elbow, or ankle, none of these
suggestions is convincing.

Clinical Features

The lesion starts as a small, painless nodule in the dermis that in paler skins
can be seen to be erythematous. Beginning in the deeper parts of the dermis or
the subcutaneous tissue, the nodule enlarges, looking rather like a painless car-
buncle, and becomes fluctuant. After a few weeks the center breaks down to
form a small ulcer, from which a gelatinous serosanguinous material can be
expressed. Even in this early period, a swab inserted into the ulcer to clean
away the necrotic material will demonstrate that the edge of the ulcer is undermined to a surprising degree, thus demonstrating that the necrosis in the lower
part of the dermis is much greater in diameter than is the overlying ulcer (Figure 7-1). From now on, the necrosis and the ulcer steadily extend. The patient

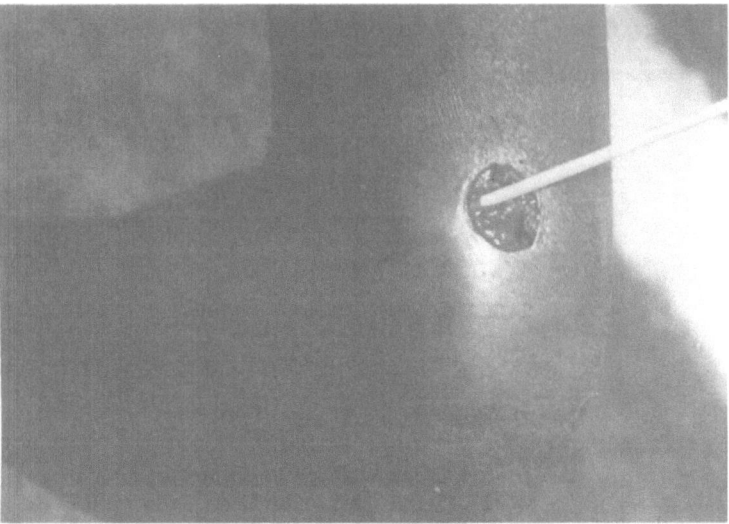

FIGURE 7-1   Mycobacterium ulcerans infection. Note swelling and a punched-out
ulcer that is undermined to a depth of more than a centimeter.

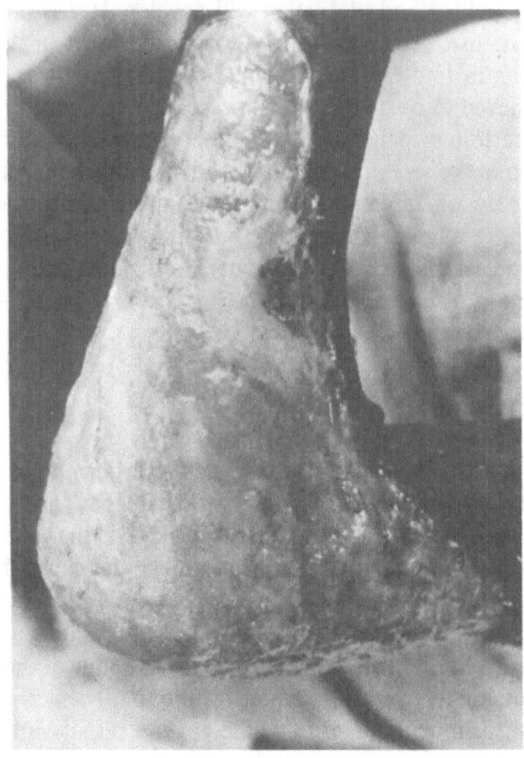

a

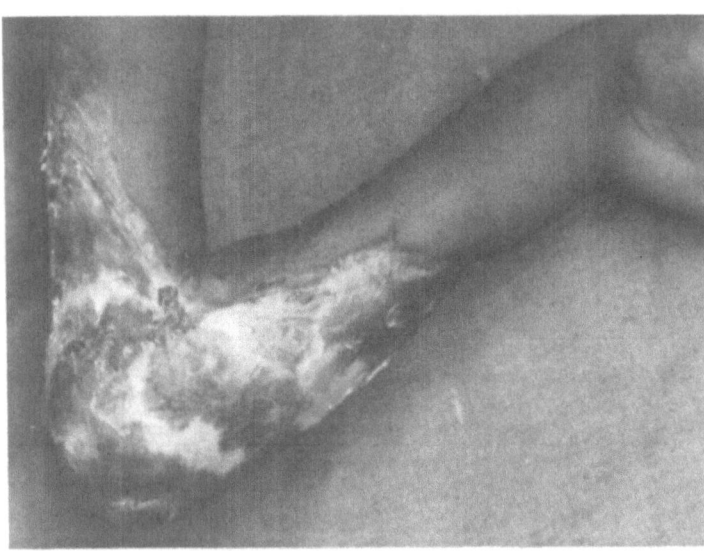

b

FIGURE 7-2   a. Mycobacterium ulcerans. A very extensive ulcer of the elbow; this child had previously had a leg removed for a similar ulcer. b. The same ulcer after medical treatment and grafting. The arm was saved but the joint was fixed.

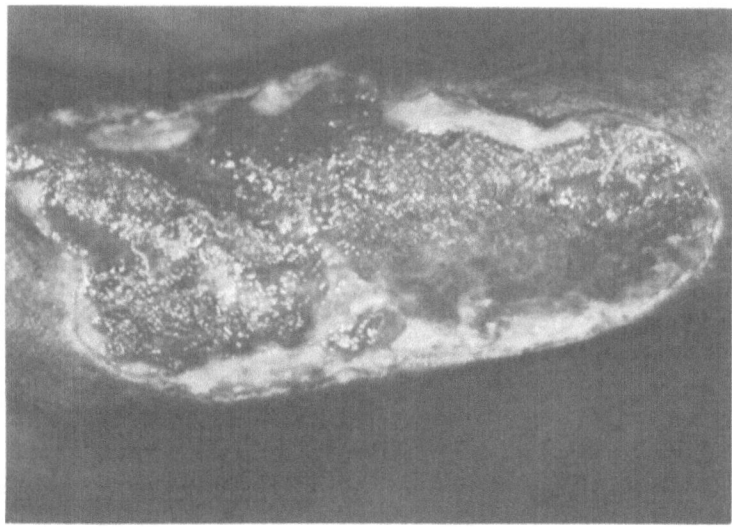

FIGURE 7-3   Undermined Buruli ulcer of the arm.

may first appear with an extremely large ulcer 10 cm or more in diameter with a necrotic base. (Figure 7-2 a, b). The ulcer is suprisingly painless, although cleaning beneath the undermined edge is rather uncomfortable. Occasionally, such large areas are undermined that other parts of the skin break down to form neighboring ulcers separated from each other by skin bridges under which a probe can be passed (Figures 7-3 to 7-5).

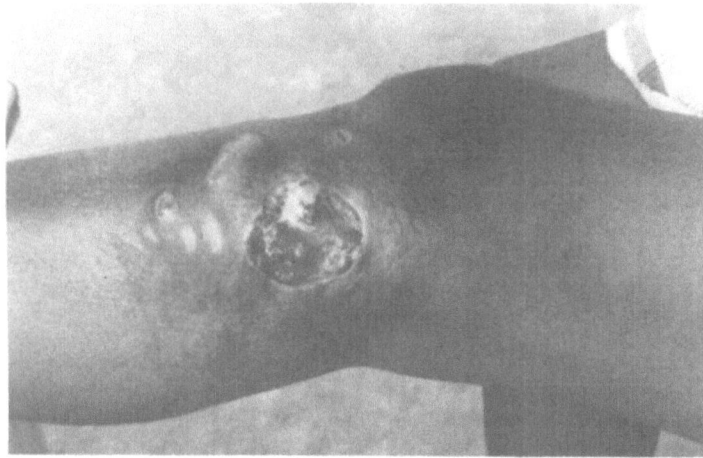

FIGURE 7-4   Buruli ulcer of the outer side of the left leg with extensive undermining of ulcer edges.

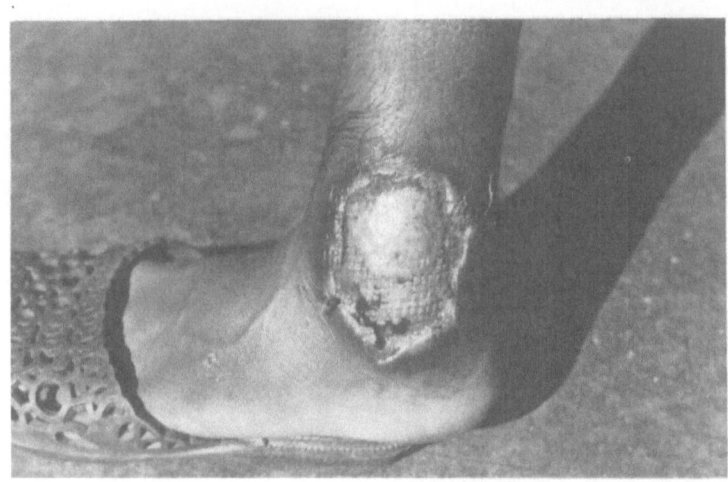

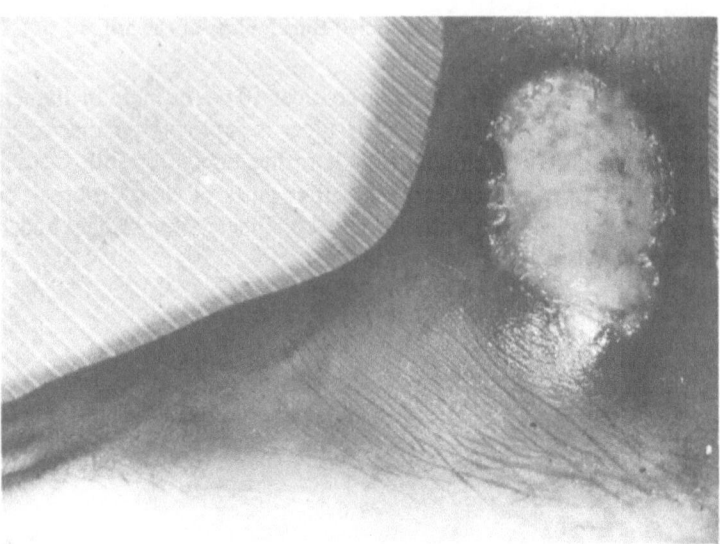

FIGURE 7-5   a. Extensive Buruli ulcer over left lateral malleous. The undermined edge is rolled in on itself. b. Same patient after treatment. The ulcer has completely healed, leaving a number of skin tags around the margin.

The patient hardly ever shows systemic symptoms; fever is rare, and lymphadenitis and lymphadenopathy are probably unknown except in association with secondary infection. Multiple lesions, arising in different parts of the body, are unusual in most countries but seem to be much more frequent in Zaire, where up to 20 percent of the cases are multiple.

A less common presentation is sometimes seen in African cases, in which the buttocks or thigh become swollen and indurated and pass through a dramatic range of discoloration until massive necrosis intervenes. It is not known whether this is a manifestation of different susceptibility in the patients or variant toxicity in the organism. In a few cases, the infection spreads along the tissue planes and even penetrates to the bone and cartilage of the joints. It is difficult to understand how this spread can be caused by an organism that prefers to grow at less than body temperature. Probably, such extension will only be seen when massive infection invades an unusually susceptible individual, one who is malnourished or has poor immunity.

Natural History

The incubation period is unknown, but as inoculation of the *M. ulcerans* into the skin of various animals usually produces lesions in four to eight weeks, the disease probably takes about the same time in humans. The nodule breaks down about six weeks after it has appeared, and the ulcer spreads steadily, usually reaching a diameter of three or more centimeters in about four to five months. It is hard to decide how many patients undergo spontaneous recovery and so do not present themselves for treatment. Sometimes, individuals are seen with an active ulcer and a scar elsewhere, which, they claim, was a similar ulcer that healed by itself. As ulcers are often seen that are spreading actively in some areas and seem to be epithelializing well in others, it is possible that spontaneous healing does occur, but patients take such a long time to improve, even with treatment, that it is thought most cases do not heal naturally. Grisly stories of amputation are not infrequent in endemic areas, where the diagnosis has only recently been recognized.

Differential Diagnosis

Any form of ulcer that has started in a tropical area always should be viewed carefully, as there are other possibilities to be excluded. Staphylococcal furuncles and carbuncles are hot and painful and easily differentiated from the cool, painless early Buruli ulcer, while pyodermatous ulcers are rarely solitary, large, or undermined. Phagedenic ulcers, which are sometimes blamed on fusospirochetes, heal rapidly when treated with metronidazole. The usually single ulcers caused by *Corynebacterium pyogenes* occur in epidemics afflicting school children and respond rapidly to a course of penicillin for one week. Ulcers due to diphtheritic organisms in the skin, so common in North Africa during World War II, seem to have disappeared almost entirely, while tuberculous ulcers (see Chapter 5) and vasculitis ulcers differ widely in clinical presentation.

The most similar lesion is probably that of pyoderma gangrenosum, but the undermining here is less extensive and the rapid improvement that usually follows even a few weeks' treatment with clofazimine (despite the absence of any mycobacteria) will soon separate these patients.

A rare condition, called Meleney's burrowing ulcer, also called synergistic bacterial gangrene, is a bacterial infection complicating surgical proceedings; it has a totally different clinical history.

Other ulcers that contain mycobacteria (Lucio's phenomenon and erythema nodosum leprosum) occur in lepromatous leprosy, but they are multiple, small, and associated with general symptoms, fever, leprosy adenitis, etc. (see Chapter 6.) Scorpion and snake bites could cause similar morphologic destruction.

Investigations

It must always be borne in mind that a chronic spreading ulcer with deeply undermined edges in a patient who either lives in or has visited the tropics is probably a Buruli ulcer. The clinical appearance is so typical that laboratory confirmation of the diagnosis is frequently an unnecessary luxury.

Bacteriology

A swab taken from the depths of the undermined pocketing may produce a positive growth on Lowenstein-Jensen medium at 32°C within three to six weeks of being set up, while tissue removed by punch biopsy from the spreading edge of the lesion (not the edge of the ulcer, which is usually necrotic and in which organisms are rarely to be found) can be processed and injected into the mouse footpad, producing a swelling of tissue within three to four weeks.

The organism is not only acid-fast, staining deeply with the Ziehl-Neelsen stain, but it can be differentiated from *M. leprae* and *M. tuberculosis* in that it is markedly Gram positive. The Bairnsdale bacillus also stains well in histology sections, as it is markedly hematoxylinophilic and shows up well with the ordinary hematoxylin and eosin stain.

Histology

This is sometimes confusing, as a biopsy of the necrotic tissue will show nothing diagnostic (except perhaps a few stained organisms), and biopsies from the spreading edge may show different forms of granuloma, from the tuberculoid with Langhans' giant cell to sections that are more suggestive of a lepromatous reaction, with foam cells and giant cells of a foreign-body type.

Before the ulcer heals, acid-fast bacilli disappear from the tissue. This is followed by regeneration, with fibroblastic proliferation leading to scar formation.

Treatment

The scattered incidence of this disease, which usually occurs in places where controlled comparison of various therapies is difficult if not impossible, has lead to diverging claims as to the efficacy of various treatments.

Systemic Treatment

In most countries, neither isonicotinic acid hydrazide nor dapsone has been of much help, and streptomycin is not recommended. The most commonly used systemic medications are rifampin (300 mg one to three times a day according to the size of the patient) either alone or in association with clofazimine (100 mg one to three times daily). Such treatment must be continue for at least six months. It is often found that the early small lesions heal satisfactorily on this routine. Larger lesions need local treatment as well.

Local Therapy

It is advisable to remove the gelatinous serosanguinous necrotic mess. This is best done by cleaning twice daily beneath the undermined edges with a swab and some form of antiseptic or astringent—eusol or Burow's solution. Care should be taken that the widespread cleansing extends in all directions. It is sometimes useful to treat the floor of the ulcer with 1 percent silver nitrate solution, if granulation tissue seems too proliferative. A silver nitrate stick moistened with water can also be used.

With this combination of systemic and local therapy it is often found that the undermined skin reattaches itself to the clean floor of the ulcer. Such adhesion will not occur if the ulcer is sited over a mobile joint (especially the knee or elbow). Such joints should be immobilized to allow healing. Discharging necrotic material will rapidly saturate the plaster, making it necessary not only to immobilize the joint but to cut a window in the plaster to permit continuing ulcer toilet (Figures 7-6a, b).

As the organism prefers to live at 32°C, heat therapy has been suggested. In its simplest form, the affected limb can be placed for several hours a day in a large box with an electric light bulb—100 watts will usually raise the circumambient air to about 40°C. Electric cradles may be used in more sophisticated areas.

Surgical Treatment

It is traditional for the surgically minded to urge widespread debridement of the ulcer edges and the necrotic material. There is conflict of opinion as to whether the unnatural enlargement of an already sizable ulcer can possibly lead to a more rapid cure. The use of pinch grafts on the ulcer will not be

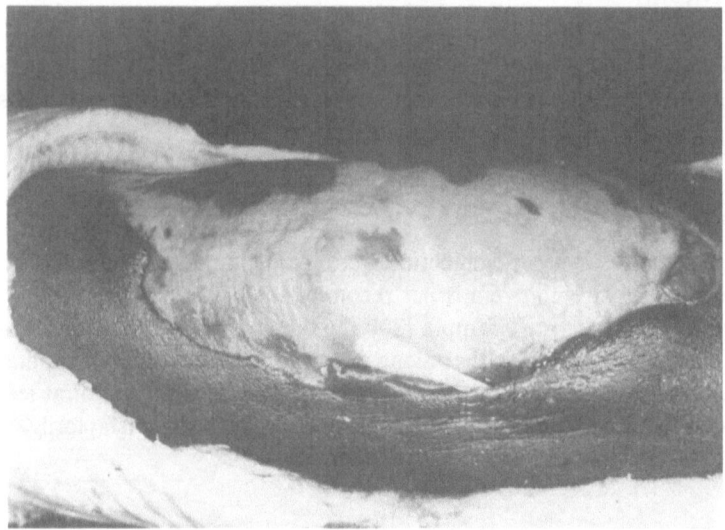

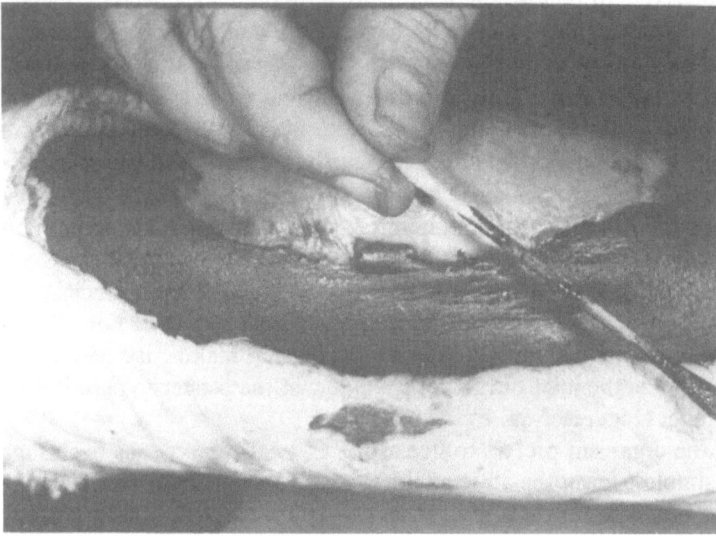

FIGURE 7-6   a,b. Buruli ulcer of the knee immobilized in plaster of Paris with a window cut to allow draining under the ulcer edge.

successful until systemic and local therapy have eliminated at least most of the pathogens, and by that time spontaneous re-epithelialization frequently will have started.

There is little doubt that a small early lesion (especially one that has not ulcerated) can be satisfactorily excised, but such lesions are rarely recognized until total excision is a practical impossibility.

The following routine is advised:

1. Immobilization of the joint with a skin window to enable ulcer toilet with eusol or Burow's solution.
2. Suitable doses of rifampin and clofazimine for at least six months.
3. As the necrosis diminishes and the ulcer floor becomes covered with healthy granulation tissue, pinch grafts may be used.
4. Excision of undermined skin should be avoided until it is certain that the above routine has not been successful (at least six months).

Follow-up

All patients should be observed for one to two years after apparent cure, since it is not unknown for a satellite ulcer to appear after treatment is stopped, probably because fibrosis around a pocket of infection has prevented a suitable therapeutic level of drug from reaching the area.

Selected Readings

Connor, DH, Lunn, HF: Buruli ulcerations: Clinical study of 38 Ugandans with mycobacterial ulcerans ulcerations. *Arch Pathol* 1966; 81:183.

Parish, LC, Millikan, LE, Witkowski, JA: Thoughts on tropical dermatology. *Int J Dermatol* 1983; 22:18.

Pettit, JHS, Rees, RJW, Marchete, NJ: Mycobacterium ulcerans infection: Clinical and bacteriologic study of cases recognized in Southeast Asia. *Br J Dermatol* 1966; 78:187.

Radford, AJ: Ulcerans ulcer: The sore that heals in vain. *Int J Dermatol* 1975; 14:422.

Ziefer, A, Connor, DH, Gibson, DW: Mycobacterium ulcerans: Infection of two patients in Liberia. *Int J Dermatol* 1981; 20:362.

CHAPTER 8

Tropical Ulcers

Many dermatoses of worldwide incidence may cause ulcers on the skin, but ulcers also develop in some diseases that occur predominantly in tropical and subtropical regions. When these are seen in temperate zones, they can cause problems in diagnosis. The clinical index (chapter 2) draws attention to a number of diseases discussed in this book that are known to cause ulceration at least sometimes during their course; diagnosis and treatment of these conditions are considered in the relevant chapters.

There remain a number of other conditions that have been studied and described in the past century. Unfortunately, sometimes the same name has been used to describe more than one picture, and the resulting confusion has led some dermatologists working in temperate zones to suspect that these conditions are not separate entities. They believe the organisms said to be the cause of such ulcers are simply secondary invaders of lesions that might have been diagnosed differently if the observers had better training in dermatology. It has been suggested that many of these lesions are associated with malnutrition, anemia, or poor hygiene and that the organisms that have been incriminated at various times do not necessarily play an etiologic role in the initiation of the disease.

Certain lesions, however, seem to be persistently associated with some of the poorer parts of the third world, and descriptions from various sources are similar enough for it to be at least possible that some of the ulcers mentioned here are individual entities.

Some Tropical Ulcers

Some writers use the words *tropical ulcer* to cover any ulcer that occurs in the tropics, but others have limited the words to an entity that is perhaps most often seen in the poorer parts of Africa and India. This is the condition discussed here. The ulcers may occur in epidemic proportions, particularly in prisons, but they are usually endemic and sporadic, most frequently affecting the legs or ankles. The lesion is usually solitary and starts with a very painful papule surrounded by a dusky areola that gives way to necrosis. The margins become somewhat indurated and the ulcerative process spreads deeply into the dermis. The base of these ulcers is covered with dirty, malodorous granulations (Figures 8-1, 8-2).

Most of the smaller ulcers resolve spontaneously within three or four months, leaving a parchmentlike scar. Some, however, become phagedenic (i.e., they start to erode extensively) and involve muscle, tendon, and bone. Such cases can remain unhealed for several years, sometimes undergoing malignant degeneration at the edge. This is one of the more common forms of cancer in certain parts of Africa.

These ulcers sometimes occur in association with other organisms, but Vincent's organisms (an association of a fusiform bacillus with the *Treponema vincenti*) are found so frequently that although there is no firm proof, this clinical picture probably occurs when Vincent's organisms invade traumatized skin of anemic or malnourished children.

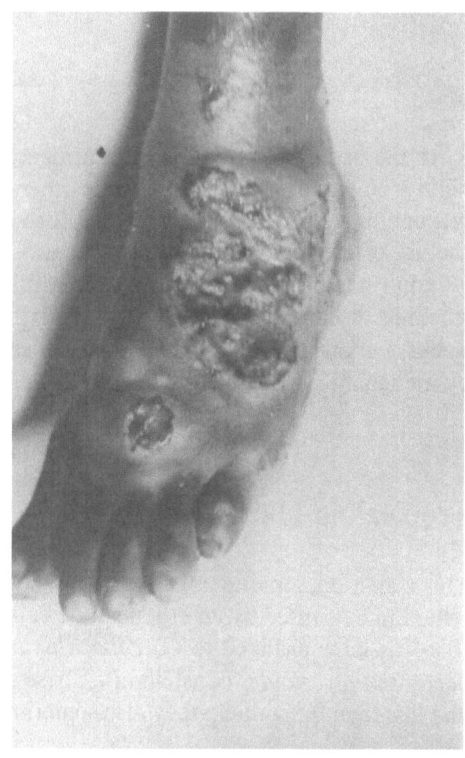

FIGURE 8-1 Ulcers and sinus tracts with purulent discharge. (Courtesy Arturo Tapia, M.D., Panama City, Panama.)

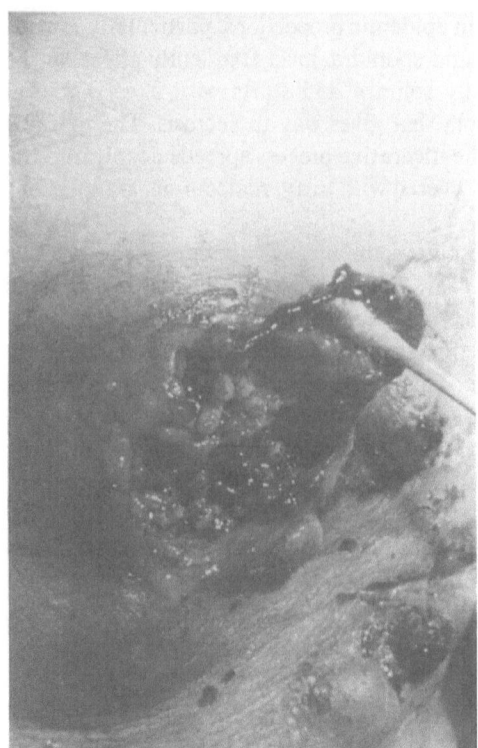

FIGURE 8-2 Ulcer contami-
nated by maggots. (Courtesy
Arturo Tapia, M.D., Panama
City, Panama.)

In the past, various forms of treatment were recommended. Systemic penicillin is effective in some cases, while others, less than 5 cm in diameter, usually
respond to a simple regimen of good food, rest, and proper hygiene. Recently,
the use of metronidazole in doses ranging up to 400 mg three times daily for
an adult has been dramatically successful in many cases. The pain and foul-
smelling discharge disappear first, and the ulcer is said to heal within two
weeks. Larger ulcers may need to be excised, especially if they are complicated
by malignant change or pseudoepitheliomatous hyperplasis.

Tropicaloid Ulcer

This condition, sometimes called mycetoid desert sore, was found by Aldo Castellani to be caused by an organism he called *Micrococcus mycetoides,* a name
that was later changed to *Coccobacillus mycetoides* and later still to *Corynebacterium mycetoides* (Castellani). These small rods are only 1 to 2 μ in length
and less than 0.5 μ thick; they also sometimes show clublike and coccoid forms.

During World War II, the condition was found to be especially prevalent in military personnel fighting in North Africa, and the ulcer has also been encountered in other parts of the Mediterranean basin as well as in northern Australia, where there is a similar climate. It differs from the Vincent form of tropical ulcer in that there are usually two or three painless, round, shallow ulcers, 1 to 2 cm in diameter, covered with a thin film of pus and often surrounded by an impetiginized dermatitis.

As it has been claimed that 60 percent of these patients also have impetigo, it is suggested that tropicaloid ulcers are simply ecthyma with a corynebacterial contaminant.

The condition clears up in two to three months without treatment, but responds faster to soap, water, and local antibacterial applications.

Diphtheritic Ulcer

Also reported during World War II in North Africa was a similar ulcer that was known to have been caused by *Corynebacterium diphtheriae*. Within a few days of the appearance of a papulopustule, there is necrotic breakdown of the epidermis. As the ulcer enlarges, a diphtheritic membrane appears on its floor, which can be removed only with difficulty. Various forms of diphtheritic paralysis (especially of the soft palate) can accompany the ulcers, which heal rapidly when antidiphtheritic serum is given. With the effective use of vaccines causing almost complete disappearance of diphtheria, these sores are probably nonexistent at present, but they will be seen again if diphtheria epidemics return to a hot, dry climate.

Veldt Sore

This is probably not an entity. The name has been used at various times for the tropical mycetoid and the diphtheritic ulcers.

Corynebacterium Pyogenes Ulcers

Corynebacterium pyogenes frequently affects farm animals but is rarely found in human beings except as a cause of respiratory infections. It has been found to affect the skin in Thailand, where a number of epidemics of skin ulcers have occurred in various schools. The children have foul-smelling lesions (usually solitary and not more than 2 cm in diameter) with an irregular outline, which contrasts with other tropical ulcers. The ulcers have a granulomatous sloughing base but do not interfere with the patient's general health. They ae surprisingly painless.

Most cases seem to be self-healing, although simple wet dressings with Burow's solution will speed things up.

Selected Readings

Bailey, H: Ulcers of the leg and their differential diagnosis. *Dermatol Tropica* 1962; 1:45.

Girolami, M, Capocaccia, L: Tropicaloid ulcers. *Dermatol Tropica* 1962; 1:78.

Kotrarjarass, R, Buddhavudhikrai, R, Sokrsongreung, S, et al: Endemic leg ulcers caused by *Corynebacterium pyogenes* in Thailand. *Int J Dermatol* 1982; 21:407.

Yesudian, P, Thambiah, AB: Metronidazole in the treatment of tropical phagednic ulcers. *Int J Dermatol* 1979; 18:755.

PART THREE

Fungal Diseases

CHAPTER 9

Tropical Tineas

Most of the fungal diseases that affect the outer layers of the skin and the hair can be seen in any part of the world. There are, however, a few that, although they may develop in temperate zones, are much more common in warmer countries. Three of these will be discussed here: tinea nigra, first clearly described in Sri Lanka, tinea imbricata, originally recognized on Oceania; and favus, the most common cause of tinea capitis in the Middle East and North Africa.

The name tinea is commonly used as a synonym for "ringworm," a dermatosis caused by keratinophilic fungi of the genera *Trichophyton, Microsporum,* and *Epidermophyton,* which have an avidity for cornified epidermis, hair, and nails.

By definition, tinea nigra is a misnomer, as the causative organism is not a dermatophyte, but the error has been perpetuated for so long that no other name is widely accepted.

Tinea Nigra

This condition, also called tinea nigra palmaris, is seen most often in Asia and South America, being relatively rare in Africa. Patients can be found in Europe and North America, where nearly 80 cases have been reported. It consists simply of black-brown macules coalescing to form an irregular polycyclic patch looking like India ink absorbed onto blotting paper. There are no scales or vesicles such as are seen in cases of true dermatophyte infection.

In Caucasians, the condition is usually golden-brown, while in darker races the condition may be black.

Etiology

The causative organism is *Cladosporium werneckii,* recently renamed *Exophiala werneckii.* It is a black, almost yeastlike fungus, somewhat like *Fonsecaea dermatiditis,* the cause of chromomycoses.

Clinical Features

Sharply marginated brown to black macules are seen on the palms or sometimes the plantar surfaces. The lesions are rarely pruritic nor are they often red. Occasionally, they can occur on the face, neck, or thorax.

Natural History

A recent account described a lesion of tinea nigra that developed on the sole of a dermatologist twenty years after he had experimentally inoculated the fungus onto the site. It is not known how long it takes for a naturally occurring disease to become visible, but as case reports of tinea nigra in young people are hard to find, it is suspected that the incubation period is probably a matter of years rather than months.

Differential Diagnosis

A junctional nevus may look the same (but it usually appears earlier in life), and malignant lentigo may also be suspected. Both of the former would not be easily scraped away.

Investigations

Microscopic examination of a KOH mount of a scraping will easily demonstrate the presence of the heavily pigmented mycelia of *Exophiala werneckii*. This grows well on Sabouraud's agar, where it produces a shiny black yeastlike colony, which is why some people group tinea nigra with the chromomycoses. Later, grey to green aerial hyphae can be seen.

If the diagnosis has not been recognized clinically and a biopsy has been taken, Gram-positive organisms may be found in the stratum corneum.

Treatment

As the infection is always very superficial, it is surprising that routine epidermal turnover does not lead to spontaneous remission of the infection. Despite its astonishing persistence, there is no reason for such a small and unimportant lesion to be treated systemically. Often after treatment and clinical cure, the organism can be recovered from the site. It can be scraped off until no further discoloration is visible, after which Whitfield's ointment should be applied twice daily for a month. Relapses with this treatment have not been reported, probably because the very long incubation period means that relapse takes many years to become clinically visible.

If the patient objects to the use of a greasy application to a lesion on the palm, benzoic acid 6 percent and salicylic acid 3 percent in 70 percent alcohol may be used instead. Other tropical treatment can be used such as clotrimazole or miconazole cream or lotion, twice daily for two weeks or econazole once daily for two weeks, but these are often no better than a keratolytic agent.

Tinea Imbricata

This is a true tinea in that it is caused by a member of the trichophyton group of fungi called *Trichophyton concentricum*. The disease has innumerable names: tinea concentricum, tinea imbricata, and Tokelau ringworm being the most frequently used.

This exotic disease affects some of the most underdeveloped countries in the world. Probably originating in Southeast Asia, it is found in the Malaysian and Australian aborigine communities, in the jungle dwellers of New Guinea, Irian Jaya, and the Amazon basin, in the Vietnamese highlands, and in many islands of the Pacific, including Samoa, Fiju, and Tokelau. It was during his visit to the Philippines that Dampier noted its distinctive appearance and described it in 1727. Curiously, it is absent from Africa and northern Australia, with a few cases found in South America.

Etiology

The causative organism is an anthropophilic dermatophyte that grows widely on the skin but is not known to invade the hair or the nails.

In countries where many races live side by side, it is rare to find tinea imbricata in any but the aborigine communities. In Malaysia, where aborigines have gradually settled into a nonnomadic rural agricultural existence, Tokelau ringworm has been dying away.

Clinical Features

Patients who have had the disease for a few years are an unforgettable sight. The skin is covered with more or less concentric rings of superficial furfuraceous scaling. As they extend, the rings finally coalesce to produce large areas of hypopigmented skin festooned with scaly circles, the whole area looking like a maritime map in which numerous islands are surrounded by depth soundings. Patient will usually agree on questioning that the condition is pruritic, but it is rare to see evidence of excoriation.

Tinea imbricata is common in childhood and early adult life and seems to be less frequent in older patients, although, of course, in such communities old age is rarer than it is elsewhere.

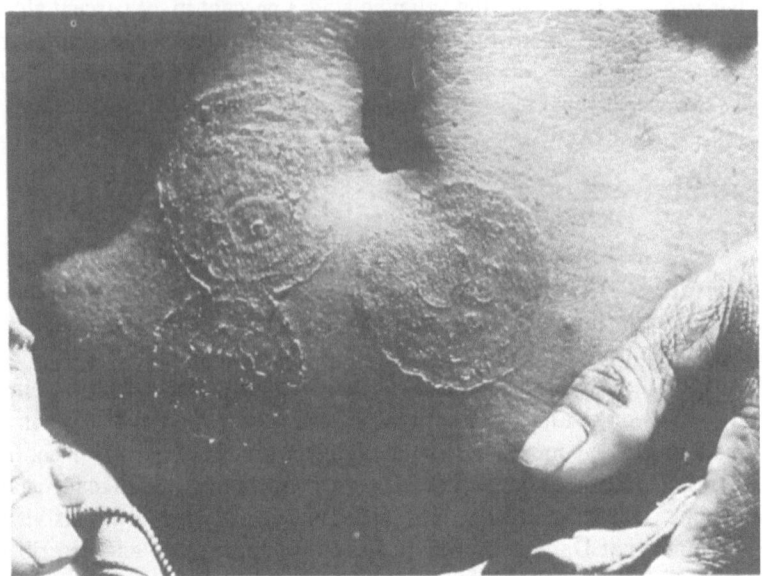

FIGURE 9-1   An early case of tinea imbricata—three lesions extending peripherally.

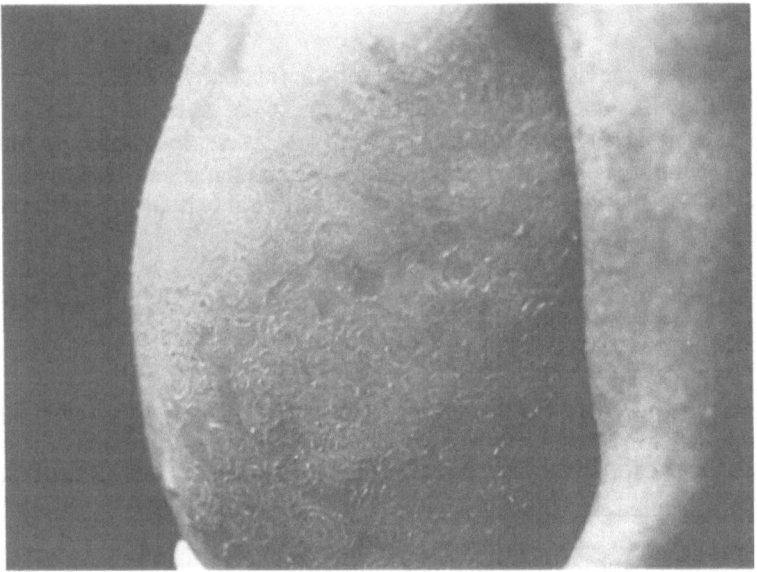

FIGURE 9-2   An extensive case of tinea imbricata; all affected skin is hypopigmented, and the few patches of normal skin have kept their color.

Natural History

Patients rarely ask for treatment while the disease is in its early stages, but experimental inoculation has shown how it starts. After seven to ten days a small red macule appears, which turns into an itchy papule that slowly extends as a circle of peripherally attached scales (Figure 9-1). With the enlargement of the original ring, new centrifugal circles start in the center, until a patch may consist of as many as ten concentric rings. The disease easily spreads to other parts of the body (most affected patients live in communities where little or no clothing is worn), and the hypopigmented lesions finally coalesce (Figure 9-2). Despite reports to the contrary, lesions can involve the face. The infection of the limbs may extend onto the sole or palm, where the typical scaliness is modified by the thicker than average palmar-plantar stratum corneum (Figure 9-3). It is thought that exposure to *T. concentricum* before the age of two offers the best means of contracting the disease. On the other hand, there is some evidence that the tendency to become infected with *T. concentricum* is due to an autosomal recessive inheritance pattern.

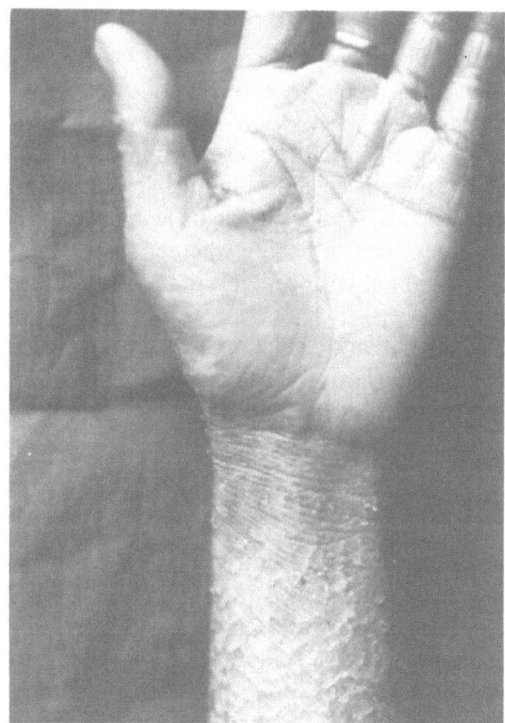

FIGURE 9-3 Extensive tinea imbricata spreading down the arm onto the palm.

Differential Diagnosis

The classical picture is unmistakable but in long-standing cases large areas of skin become so scaly that it may be confused with ichthyosis. The scales of tinea imbricata are larger and dirty-looking, and ichthyotics give a different history. A very extensive confluent tinea versicolor can sometimes look the same—the cellophane-tape test (see Appendix one) will show the true diagnosis. The test is negative in tinea imbricata.

Other forms of ringworm may have papules or vesicles at the spreading edge, neither of which is seen here.

Investigations

Scraping of the skin will produce scales full of mycelial filaments, and culture on Sabouraud's agar produces a folded, slowly growing thallus somewhat darker than *T. schoenleinii,* which it closely resembles. Microscopic examination of the culture will show branching hyphae, rarely with any spores.

Treatment

The condition responds rapidly to routine forms of antimycotic therapy. 500 mg of fine-particle griseofulvin or ketoconazole (200 mg) given daily will cause dramatic disappearance of the lesions in 10 to 14 days; Whitfield's ointment, econazole, miconazole, and clotrimazole cream or lotion have all been successful, but there is an almost immediate relapse in most cases as soon as treatment has stopped. Treatment should continue for six weeks to reduce the relapse rate. It is open to debate whether these patients, living as they do in a style that would not be acceptable in the Western world, have relapsed or have been reinfected.

Many patients dislike using greasy applications over large areas of skin, and in Malaysia they prefer to use Whitfield's lotion—a mixture of benzoic acid 6 percent and salicylic acid 3 percent in methylated spirit.

Favus

Most forms of tinea capitis are produced by fungi whose spores invade or surround hair, which, as a result, becomes fragile and breaks off at or near the scalp level. This causes circular patches of slightly scaly but otherwise uninflamed skin. A rare complication known as kerion can cause residual scarring, but otherwise tinea capitis resolves completely, leaving a normal head of hair. The condition undergoes natural remission at puberty. Although it is reported in a few postmenopausal women, it is almost unknown in older people. In contradistinction to typical tinea capitis, favus, also called tinea favosa, shows no tendency to spontaneous resolution and spreads slowly but inexorably over the scalp, leaving a permanently atrophic alopecia.

The condition, once epidemic in the United States and Eastern Europe, is very common in the Middle Eastern countries and Central America, but is rare in black Africa. The disease seems to be more at home in the arid subtropical regions than in the equatorial rain forests. In Iraq, 70 percent of all tinea capitis is favus.

Etiology

Trichophyton schoenleinii is a highly infectious fungus that spreads easily from child to child, particularly those living or working in cramped quarters. As there is no tendency for remission, most hairs of the scalp are infected throughout their length, so pieces snipped off by a barber will contain spores that will infect others who share a comb, a cap, or a bed. In fact, *T. schoenleinii* can live in these cut hairs for even 20 or 30 years. Fortunately, in the Middle East and North Africa it is socially acceptable to shave children's heads. This not only diminishes the child's chance of having pediculosis capitis but reduces the likelihood of favus.

Clinical Features

This is the most socially crippling disease produced by a dermatophyte. It is not unusual to find communities where more than half the residents have scarred baldness. Typically, an established active case has patches of wrinkled atrophy mixed with widespread yellowish crusts which are firmly attached to the skin by hairs that have not yet fallen out (Figure 9-4a,b). It is among these crusts that the diagnostic scutula are seen, caused by mycelial overgrowth in the stratum corneum, producing an accumulation of keratinized and parakeratotic cells. This is attached centrally to the underlying epidermis but is peripherally detached where it curls away from the skin to give a saucer-shaped crust, producing a characteristic mousy odor and classically being described as cup-shaped. In a large series of cases from Iran only about half the patients had these scutula—their presence is a manifestation of long-standing active disease but their absence in early cases does not impeach the diagnosis.

Natural History

Spores probably penetrate the hairs at scalp level, and mycelia grow in each direction. At this early stage, invasion of the hair root and follicle causes minute red puncta to appear at the follicle mouth, and foci of follicular erythema

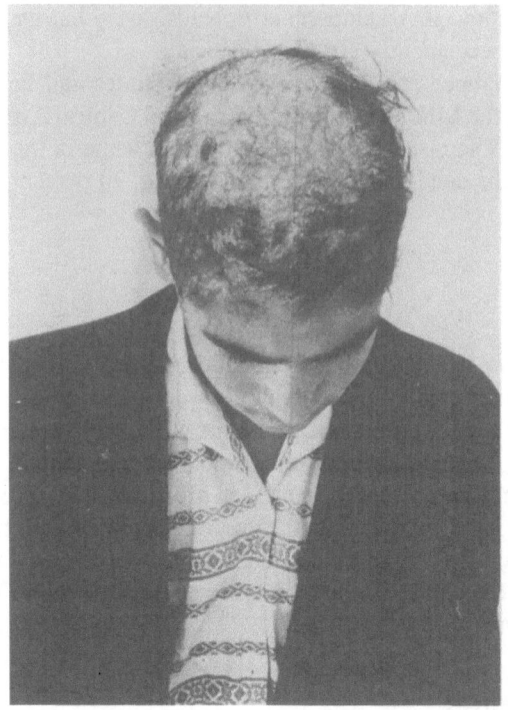

a

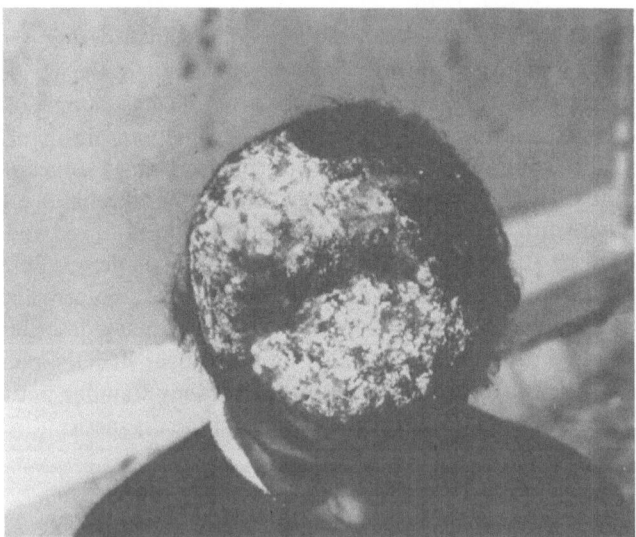

b

FIGURE 9-4   a. Extensive favus. In a widespread area of cicatricial alopecia, scattered patches of cursting persist. b. Marked crusting in an Egyptian man with favus. (Courtesy Mohsen Soliman, M.D., Cairo, Egypt.)

spread over the scalp, matting together the hairs, which take on a lusterless appearance. As the disease extends, crusts and, later, scutula develop, which, if removed, leave moist erythematous puncta in the denuded epidermis. Finally, as the hair follicles are destroyed and the alopecia spreads across the scalp, the crusts loose their yellow color and have been graphically described as being the shade of old mortar—a substance they resemble in dryness and friability. If left untreated for many years, the condition slowly subsides, leaving an extensive atrophy with islands of normal skin from which grow hairs that have managed to avoid infection.

Frequently, the edges of the scalp have remained exempt from this process, and the patient has a circular fringe of normal hair around the alopecia.

There is considerable itching on the scalp during the active stages. As a result of scratching, infection spreads via the nails to the glabrous skin. When the fingers are involved, the infection starts subungually and looks indistinguishable from other types of tinea unguium, while on the limbs and trunk T. schoenleinii occasionally produces lesions of tinea circinata with a spreading vesicular edge. More commonly vesicles are not seen, scaling predominates, and scutula develop. It is surprising how many patients with long-standing active disease never produce lesions other than on the scalp.

Differential Diagnosis

An atrophic alopecia studded with yellow, saucer-shaped crusts is easily recognizable, but in the earliest stages the scattered follicular erythema may be blamed on bacterial infection and the diagnosis will only become obvious with time.

Other causes of cicatricial alopecia (lupus erythematosus, lichen planus) are not so scaly in their active phases, while a history of x-ray therapy will accompany the atrophy that follows excessive irradiation of the scalp.

On some occasions, people with favus may have a diffuse scaliness of the scalp that can be confused with dandruff or seborrheic dermatitis, in which case the hair must be examined for evidence of infection.

Investigations

The diagnosis is most easily made by examining the hair under the Wood's light (see Appendix one), as hairs affected by favus will fluoresce a typical grey-green. If such hairs are removed and examined under the microscope, the fungus will be seen. It is an endothrix whose large spores are arranged in chains among the mycelial elements. The feature that differentiates T. schoenleinii from all other types of tinea capitis is the collection of rows of small air-bubbles, which can be recognized by their varying sizes as being different from the spores of uniform diameter.

If hair clippings are transferred to Sabouraud's agar, a slowly growing folded white colony will develop that microscopically shows hyphae with a form of branching in which the growing ends expand to look rather like moose antlers. These are called favic chandeliers.

A biopsy taken from the scalp during the active phase will show an inflammatory lesion of the follicle containing foreign-body giant cells, many plasma cells, hyphae, and spores. When the disease is burnt out, sections will show fibrosis at right angles to the epidermis as the only remains of the hair follicle.

Treatment

Ketoconazole 200 mg daily or grisofulvin 500 mg for an adult, with smaller doses for smaller patients, is the preferred treatment. The problem, however, is to determine a suitable duration of therapy. As infected hairs may grow almost indefinitely, if treatment is stopped after three to four months, living spores from the terminal portion of the hair will soon reinfect unprotected hair at scalp level.

The following routine must be insisted on for both men and women:

1. The scalp must be shaved completely at the start of treatment.
2. Suitable doses of ketoconazole or griseofulvin are administered for four weeks.
3. Twenty-five days after the start of treatment the scalp must be shaved again.
4. One month after the end of medication, when the hairs are regrowing, they should be carefully examined under the Wood's light and, in the unlikely case that there are still a few showing fluorescence, they may be removed manually and the patient is cured.

In those parts of the world where favus is endemic, local authorities should be encouraged to treat all the affected members of a community at the same time. This, with any luck, will ensure that reinfection from the neighbors is kept to a minimum.

Selected Readings

Ajello, L: The black yeasts as disease agents: historical perspective. Proceedings of the Fourth International Congress on the mycoses, PAHO publication No. 356, June 1977.

Blank, H: Tinea nigra—a 20 year incubation period? *J Am Acad Dermatol* 1979; 1:49.

Castellani, A, Chalmers, AJ: *Manual of Tropical Medicine.* New York, William Wood and Co., 1910.

Conti-Diaz, IA, Civila, E, Asconegui, F: Treatment of superficial and deep-seated mycoses with oral ketoconazole. *Int J Dermatol* 1984; 23:207.

Khan, A, McIver, FA: A case of tinea nigra palmaris from Charleston, South Carolina. JSC Med Assoc 1980; 76:464.

Miles, WJ, Branom, WT, Frank, SB: Tinea nigra. *Arch Dermatol* 1964; 94:203.

Pettit, JHS: Griseofulvin and favus. *Br J Dermatol* 1962; 74:179.

Ravine, D, Turner, KJ, Alpers, MP: Genetic inheritance of susceptibility to tinea imbricata. *J Med Genet* 1980; 17:342.

CHAPTER 10

Chromomycosis

Early in the twentieth century, the term *chromoblastomycosis* came into being and was used to cover all skin disease caused by pathogenic fungi that produced pigmented spores. In the course of time, the name changed to chromomycosis, and it is now used to denote a dermal infection found predominantly in the tropics. Pigmented cells of *Exophiala werneckii* can infect the epidermis, causing tinea nigra (see Chapter 9), while similar organisms occasionally produce internal abscesses or even infections of the brain. These conditions will not be discussed here.

Chromomycosis occurs in the tropical parts of the Americas, in India, Africa, and Southeast Asia, and is sometimes recognized in temperate climates (Europe, Taiwan, Japan, or Australia), usually in patients who have acquired the disease elsewhere.

Etiology

There is considerable confusion about the nomenclature of organisms involved in this disease. *Phialophora, Cladosporium, Fonsecaea,* and *Hormodendrum,* are all names that have been used at various times and seem to be interchangeable, while the *Exophiala werneckii* (also known as *Cladosporium werneckii*) does not invade the dermis. It is recommended that the name *Fonsecaea* be used for those organisms (*F. pedrosi, F. compacta,* and *F. verucosa*) that usually cause chromomycosis and that the names *Phialophora, Cladosporium,* and *Hormodendrum* be consigned to oblivion.

As these organisms can be found in decaying wood, soil, and vegetable debris, the disease most commonly affects agricultural workers, farmers, and gardeners, who develop lesions on the limbs as the result of traumatic inoculation.

Clinical Features

Although it is believed that inoculation is the invariable precursor of the infection, the spread of the lesion is so slow that when the patient finally gets around to seeking advice the precipitating trauma has often been forgotten.

The classical picture of chromomycosis is of a papilliferous warty lesion. It can take several forms: a spreading warty granuloma or a reddish-brown plaque occasionally studded with foul-smelling intraepidermal abscesses. The dry warty lesions are rarely painful unless they have ulcerated and become secondarily infected (Figures 10-1 to 10-5).

The infection may spread deep enough to involve the lymphatics, and sometimes the nodules extend up the limb in a sporotrichoid manner to produce a granulomatous and fibrotic inflammation of the lymph nodes.

Natural History

As most patients seek medical assistance only after the disease has been present for many years, it is difficult to determine the incubation period, but a case reported from Tacoma, Washington, showed diagnosable lesions on the hands only 16 months after the patient stumbled on a macadam driveway.

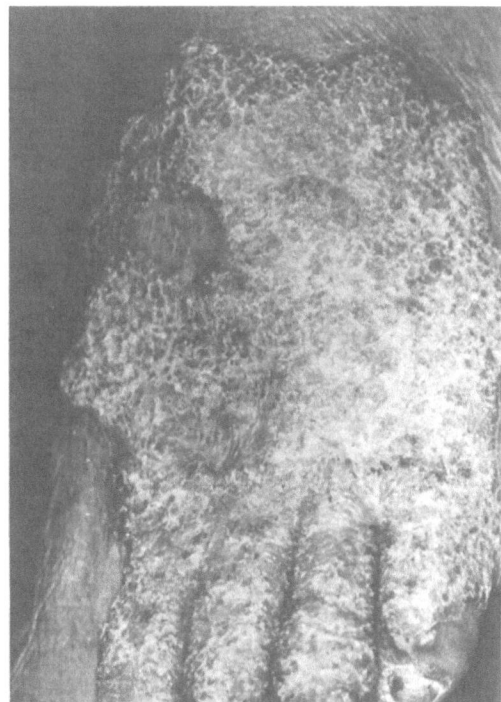

FIGURE 10-1 Dry verrucosus infiltration of dorsum of foot.

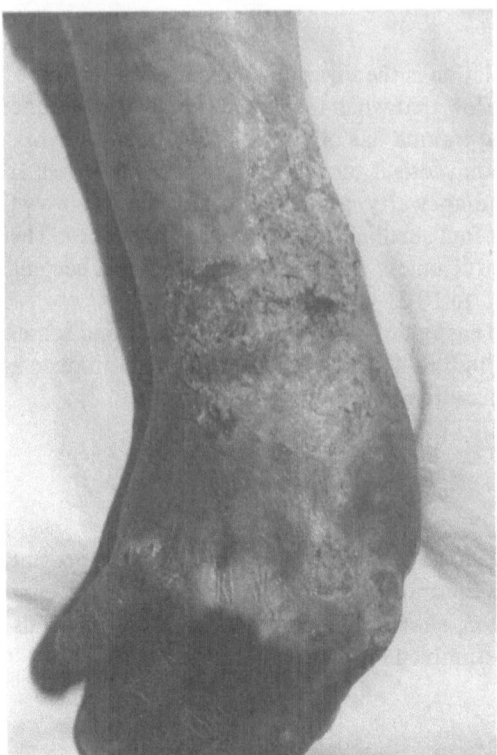

Slowly, the dermal granuloma and the warty proliferation extend in a mixture of scarring and hypertrophy that can cover the whole limb, although more often the plaque is only a few centimeters in diameter. In view of the extent that these lesions may attain, it is suspected that spontaneous resolution does not occur; there are no persuasive accounts of spontaneous recovery.

Not surprisingly, in such a chronic infection that spreads not only in the dermis and subcutaneous tissue but also to the lymphatic channels, the final stages may be complicated by a marked hyperplasia sometimes called lymphostasis verrucosa or mossy foot.

Differential Diagnosis

The classical combination of warty hyperkeratosis, papillomatosis, and scarring is fairly easy to recognize, the most likely confusion being with tuberculosis verrucosa cutis, which tends to affect the same parts of the body and to extend equally slowly. In the early stages, a small warty papule is often mistaken for a verruca vulgaris both by the patient and the physician. The lupoid form of

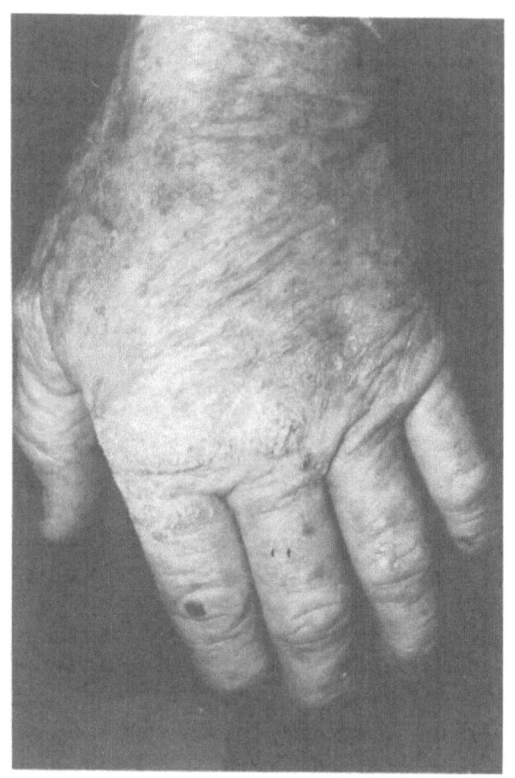

FIGURE 10-3 Scattered warty lesions and dermatitis easily confused with verruca vulgaris and hand dermatitis. (Courtesy Graeme Beardmore, M.B., Brisbane, Australia.)

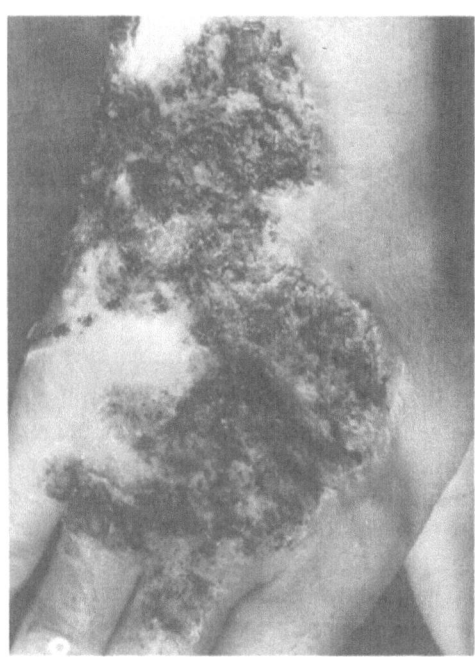

FIGURE 10-4 Extensive infection of the hand. (Courtesy Institute of Dermatology, Chinese Academy of Medical Sciences, Jiangsu, People's Republic of China.)

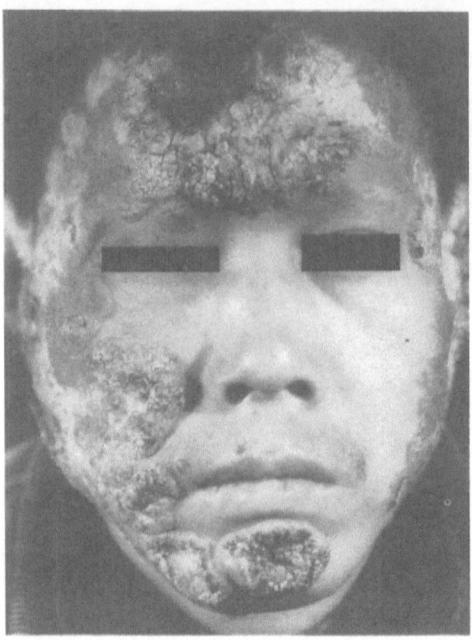

FIGURE 10-5 Verruca growth and ulceration of several years' duration on a Chinese man. (Courtesy Institute of Dermatology, Chinese Academy of Medical Sciences, Jiangsu, People's Republic of China.)

leishmaniasis rarely affects the same sites and is usually preceded by a recognizable acute leishmaniasis.

If the scarring is extensive, the later stages of syphilis or yaws may be mimicked.

Lesions with extensive abscess formation have been confused with North American blastomycosis, but they are usually differentiable as they occur in widely differing geographic sites.

Hypertrophic skin that is centrally ulcerated may be confused with a squamous or basal cell carcinoma and needs a biopsy to clarify the problem.

Investigations

The organisms causing chromomycosis live in the dermis. It is impossible to obtain samples by scraping the epidermis; if the organisms are to be recognized and cultured, it is necessary to examine material either from the discharge of any complicating abscess or from a biopsy. It is not always easy to grow, but if a culture can be successfully established, each of the *Fonsecaea* will produce soft raised black colonies that can be differentiated from each other only by experienced mycologists.

The causative organisms can more easily be demonstrated by recognizing their presence in a biopsy that has been sectioned and stained with hematoxylin and eosin. The basic pathology is of a tuberculoid granuloma, usually in the upper dermis, where the overlying epidermis has been stimulated to a marked pseudoepitheliomatous overgrowth. In the older cases, chronic fibrosis is found between the granulomata. This combination of histologic features is not in itself diagnostic, but fortunately the diagnosis is facilitated by the presence of golden-brown, thick-walled, septate fungal cells, which are most commonly seen in the Langhans' cells. These spores, rarely more than 5 μ in diameter, stand out in the section because of the golden-brown color of their cell wall, which is markedly thicker than any other cell wall in the neighboring tissue.

Treatment

By far the most successful method of curing small lesions is for them to be thoroughly excised.

For larger lesions systemic therapy is needed, but none of these is regularly successful.

Amphotericin B (50 mg injected intralesionally once a week for several months) or fluorcytosine (given orally 150 mg/kg in three divided doses each day) may both be tried; griseofulvin is completely ineffective.

The broad-spectrum antifungal drug ketoconazole, given 200 mg daily for at least three months, seems at least as successful as other therapies. It is also easier to administer, probably has less severe side effects, and is just as expensive. The drug should not, however, be given during pregnancy.

An ingenious form of therapy has been reported from Japan in which the large scaly plaques are treated by local heat therapy using an electric bed-warmer with a surface temperature of 46°C. Either this or a benzene pocket warmer can be used if all else fails, but treatment will need to be continued for several months.

Many apparently cured cases have been known to relapse, but if the recurrence is small it can be satisfactorily excised.

Selected Readings

Carrion, AL: Chromoblastomycosis and related infections. New concepts, differential diagnosis, and nomenclatorial implications. *Int J Dermatol* 1975; 14:27.

Creva-Paz, SA: Chromomicosis. *Dermatol Rev Mex* 1969; 13:139.

Fan, J, and Tsao, KL: Chromoblastomycosis. *Far East Med J* 1969; 5:151.

McGinnis, MR; Chromoblastomycosis and phaeohyphomycosis: New concepts, diagnosis and mycology. *J Am Acad Dermatol* 1983; 8:1.

Tagami, H, Ginoza, M, Imaizumi, S, et al: Successful treatment of chromoblastomycosis with topical heat therapy. *J Am Acad Dermatol* 1984; 10:615.

Vollum, DI: Chromomycosis: A review. *Br J Dermatol* 1977; 96:454.

Chapter 11

Madura Foot and Other Mycetomas

In the middle of the nineteenth century, physicians, especially in India, recognized a number of somewhat similar clinical conditions, all of which were associated with sinuses discharging pus in which various colored granules could be detected. Initially, it was believed that all these grains consisted of aggregates of fungi, and the term *mycetoma* came into being. Later, it was discovered that of the many different organisms involved some were true fungi (eumycetes) while others, the actinomycetes, are now considered to be intermediate between fungi and bacteria. These organisms infect the subcutaneous tissue and produce a number of slightly different clinical appearances, including Madura foot, which was described, not for the first time, in 1842 in the *Madurai Dispensary Reports* in the *Indian Army Medical Reports.* If any eponymous name is to be used, the condition should by rights be called the Madurai foot, but it is probably too late to alter an established misnomer.

Although Madura foot is most commonly seen in the tropics (India, Southeast Asia, Mexico, Brazil, and Africa), patients have acquired the disease as far north as California and Bulgaria and as far south as Australia.

Etiology

With the passing years, many members of the eumycete family have been recognized as causing Madura foot. Other cases, clinically indistinguishable, are caused by some of the more exotic actinomycetes, which produce white-yellow granules in the mucopurulent discharge. The eumycetes more frequently produce brown or black granules.

The condition is usually seen in men, perhaps because in most tropical areas they form the body of agricultural workers, and the condition is probably always the result of a penetrating wound. The disease is not known to spread from person to person or from animal to human.

Clinical Features

Madura Foot

When the condition is fully established, the diagnosis is unmistakable. The disease starts as a painless nodule that enlarges, softens, and breaks down (Figure 11-1). Other nodules and fistulae develop nearby, and swelling of both dorsal and plantar surfaces of the foot may be so severe that the toes can no longer make contact with the ground. The infection spreads deeply to the muscle and bone. The consequent periostitis, osteomyelitis, and osseous absorption lead to a dramatic and disabling deformity, which is surprisingly painless (Figure 11-2).

The epidermal hyperplasia seen in the chromomycoses does not occur in Madura foot. The epidermis between the discharing sinuses is usually normal, although it is sometimes possible to see a granulomatous proliferation blocking and surrounding the mouths of the sinuses.

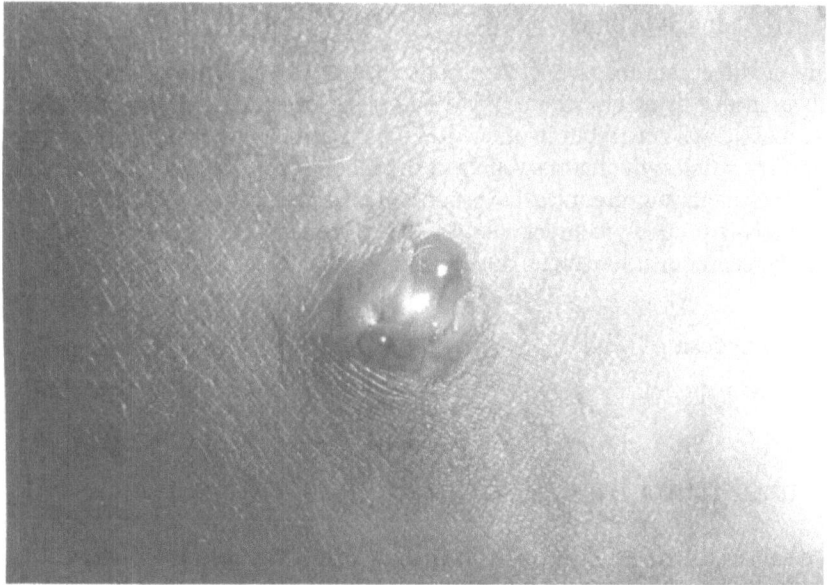

FIGURE 11-1   Painless nodule with purulent discharge in a year-old boy. (Courtesy Ramon Ruiz-Maldonado, M.D., Mexico City, Mexico.)

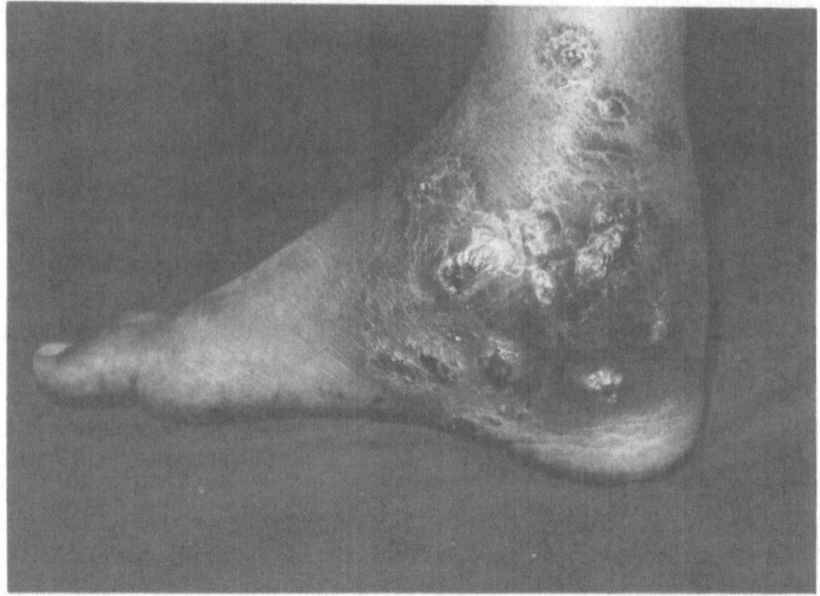

FIGURE 11-2   Ulcers and sinus tracts involving the bone in a fourteen-year-old Mexican boy. (Courtesy Ramon Ruiz-Maldonado, M.D., Mexico City, Mexico.)

Other Deep Mycetomas

Any of the organisms that cause Madura foot may, of course, penetrate the subcutaneous tissue elsewhere. If the hand is involved, deformities of the bone and muscle will occur, but in other sites the diagnosis is often difficult to establish if the painless fluctuant swelling of the skin has not yet started to discharge and the diagnostic granules have not revealed themselves. The difficulty of diagnosis is probably compounded by the infrequent incidence of the disease and the consequent low index of suspicion, especially in nonendemic areas.

Actinomycosis

See chapter 13.

Natural History

It is believed that Madura foot invariably follows a penetrating wound into subcutaneous tissue, and few cases are seen in patients who are not in the habit of walking and working barefoot. There are widely differing reports concerning

FIGURE 11-3 Sole of foot studded with sinus tracts and ulcers in a Malaysian man.

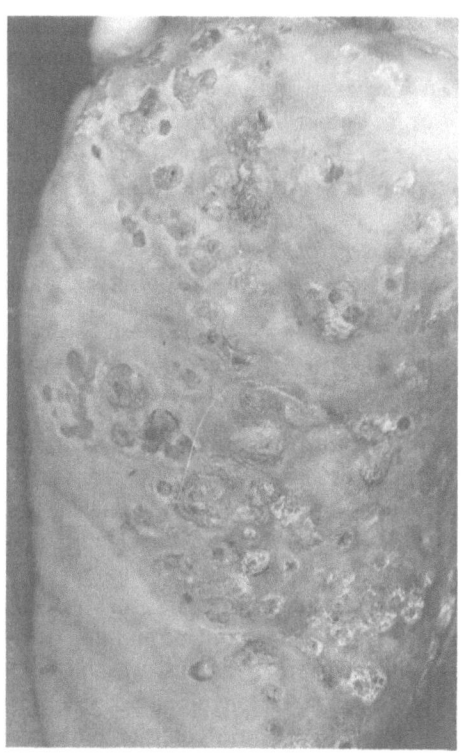

the incubation period. In a few patients, the lesion starts less than six months after trauma has occurred, but in many cases the disease is not shown to a doctor for 20 to 30 years, probably because the combination of nodules, pustules, multiple sinus tracts, fibrosis, and muscle and bone destruction is painful only if a secondary bacterial infection has invaded the damaged tissue.

There is no tendency to spontaneous cure. Slowly but surely, people with Madura foot are increasingly immobilized by appalling deformity of the limb (Figure 11-3). Infections elsewhere are hardly less troublesome.

Differential Diagnosis

A deep mycetoma is not a specific reaction to an individual organism. It is a nonspecific reaction to chronic infection of subcutaneous tissue. In the early stages, it may be hard to differentiate a mycetoma from a swollen foot caused by any bacterial or mycobacterial osteomyelitis, but bacterial infection is usually associated with fever and pain while mycobacterial osteitis (*M. tubercu-*

losis or *M. leprae*) usually accompanies other signs of the causative disease. The diagnosis is established by demonstration of the grains in the mycetoma-tous discharge or biopsy material.

Some authorities do not attempt to differentiate these mycetomas from acti-nomycosis, but it is therapeutically helpful to separate the two conditions. *Actinomyces israelii* is an anaerobic organism that spreads to the subcutaneous tissue from an underlying lesion, while mycetoma is invariably the result of inoculation from outside.

Botryomycosis (see Chapter 14) may also mimic a mycetoma clinically.

Investigations

When Madura foot is fully established, the appearance is so typical that investigations are hardly necessary. In any case, the number of organisms that may be involved and the wide range of culture media and techniques necessary to grow them usually prohibit sucessful recognition of the causative agent in the average third-world clinic. If such attempts are made, it must be remembered that granules should not be transferred to a suitable culture medium (Littman's ox-gall agar or Sabouraud's agar without cycloheximide) until they have been removed from the pus, washed in sterile water, and crushed to liberate the spores from the engulfing accretion that has collected around them.

The eumycetes most commonly recognized are:

Allescheria boydii	white granules
Cephalosporium falciforme	yellowish granules
Phialophora jeanselmei	yellow-brown granules
Madurella mycetomi	
or	brown-black granules
Madurella grisea	

The various form of actinomycetes involved include:

Nocardia braziliensis
Streptomyces madurae
Streptomyces somaliensis

These all produce yellow-white granules.

This is not a complete list, and if other organisms are isolated, it does not mean that the diagnosis necessarily has to be reconsidered.

There is usually little reason to take a biopsy from a Madura foot, but if it is done, grains will be seen surrounded by polymorphonuclear leukocytes, his-tocytes, and fibrocytes, all trying rather unsuccessfully to limit the infection.

Treatment

Less than 40 years ago, it was believed that potassium iodide was the only possible treatment, either orally (in increasing doses until iodism developed) or locally, following curettage of the sinuses. If that did not help, amputation was the only other method of eradicating the disease.

Since that time, the picture has improved somewhat, and many cases of Madura foot have responded to oral medication. More frequent isolation of the causative organism has shown that while lesions caused by *Nocardia* or *Streptomyces* respond fairly well to various drugs, the eumycetomas are much more resistant to therapy, either because they are not sensitive to available drugs or, equally possible, the grains are relatively impermeable to what seems in vitro to be a suitable medication.

As the actinomyces are not true fungi, it is not surprising that cotrimoxazole (two tablets daily for six months and then one daily for a further two years) has been found to be successful. This may be supplemented by dapsone (100 mg daily) or streptomycin in doses suitable for the size of the patient.

The eumycetes are less susceptible to such regimens, and intralesional injections of amphotericin B may be used. More recently, ketoconazole (200 mg twice daily for many months) has sometimes been effective.

The other deep mycetomas are no easier to treat systemically, but their sites often make it necessary to contemplate eradication of the whole lesion by excision, amounting even to amputation of foot.

Selected Readings

Barnetson, RSC, Milne, LJR: Mycetoma. *Br J Dermatol* 1978; 99:227.

Klokke, A, Swamidasan, G, Anguli, R, Verghese, A: The causal agents of mycetoma in South India *Trans R Soc Trop Med Hyg* 1968; 62:509.

Kotrajaras, R: Mycetoma. A review of seventeen cases seen at the Institute of Dermatology, Bangkok, Thailand. *J Dermatol* 1981; 8:133.

Magana, M: Mycetoma. *Int J Dermatol* 1984; 23:221.

Palestine, R, Rogers, R: Diagnosis and treatment of mycetoma. *J Am Acad Dermatol* 1982; 6:107.

Valabinoff, VA, Madurafuss durch nocardia asteroides. *Castellania* 1977; 5:91.

Zaias, N, Taplin, D, Rebell, G: Mycetoma. *Arch Dermatol* 1969; 99:215.

CHAPTER 12

Sporotrichosis

This deep fungus infection can be found anywhere in the world and is not particularly common in any one area. Its incidence bears no relationship to race or skin color. Men are predominantly infected, the disease generally occurring in the 20- to 50-year age group and more frequently affecting farmers, miners, construction workers, and gardeners. In one well-recorded epidemic, some 3,000 gold-miners in South Africa acquired the disease from infected wooden pitprops. It may be seen not only in humans, but also in a wide number of animals, including rats, cats, dogs, fowl, donkeys, horses, and camels.

Etiology

The offending agent is *Sporothrix* (formerly *Sporotrichum*) *schenckii*, aptly honoring Benjamin Schenck, who first described the disease in 1898. The organism is diphasic and aerobic, growing at room temperature on Sabouraud's agar in as little as five days and producing whitish colonies that rapidly change to become leathery, heaped-up, and brown or black. Smears show hyphae with lateral branches and pyriform conidia.

The organism is somewhat comparable to those causing chromomycosis, as it tends to grow on decaying vegetation, timber, straw, or sphagnum moss. It can sometimes be detected in soil or in living vegetation. As in the cases of chromomycosis, the infection usually follows local penetrating trauma although transmission is generally from the soil, zoonotic methods are conceivable.

Clinical Features

When the skin is infected, lesions occur at the site of trauma. Sometimes, the infection remains localized, but more often the disease spreads up along the lymphatic system to produce the classical sporotrichoid picture of a primary ulcerated and crusting granuloma with more recent lesions developing over the lymphatics and, especially, at the sites of the draining regional lymph nodes.

An infection on the foot, for example, may be associated with others on the calf and in the popliteal space and even ascend to the inguinal nodes, which, in the later stages, also develop soft ulcerating granulomata (Figures 12-1 to 12-5).

Natural History

In contrast to chromomycosis, lesions appear on the skin only a few days after the initial inoculation. Nodules and crusts develop that, frequently being asymptomatic, may be neglected for a considerable time. If the patient is reasonably successful at combating the infection, the lesion may remain fixed or localized indefinitely, in which case red, scaling plaques, verrucous lesions, or even the appearance of pyoderma may develop.

More frequently seen is the cutaneous lymphatic form, in which a chain of

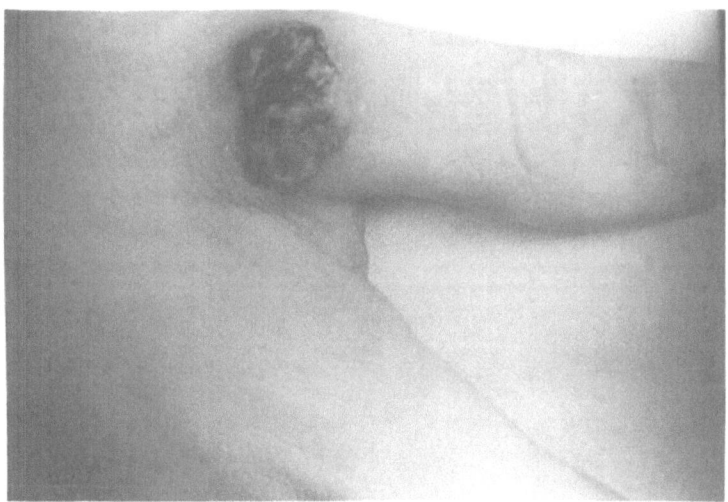

FIGURE 12-1   Chancriform lesion on the thumb. (Courtesy Arturo Tapia, M.D., Panama City, Panama.)

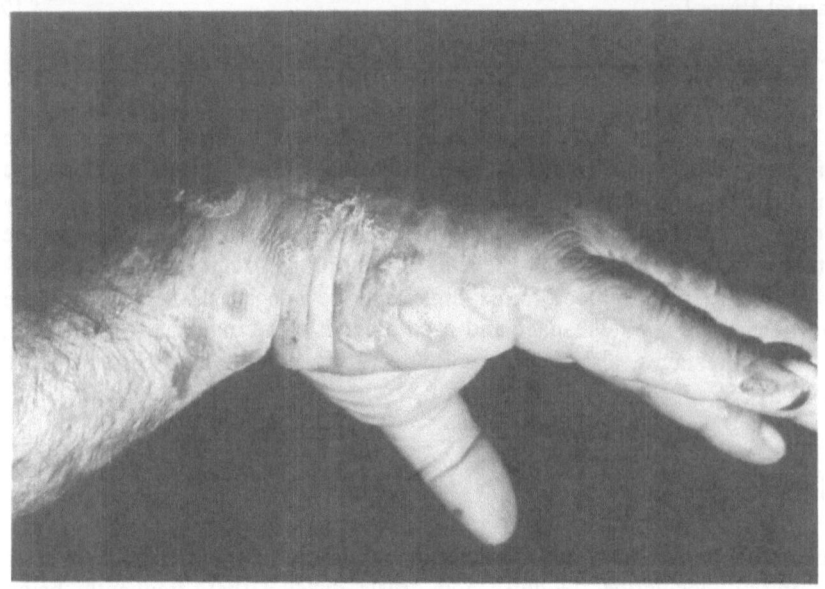

FIGURE 12-2 Extension of the crusted granulomatous lesions on the hand and wrist. (Courtesy Graeme Beardmore, M.B., Brisbane, Australia.)

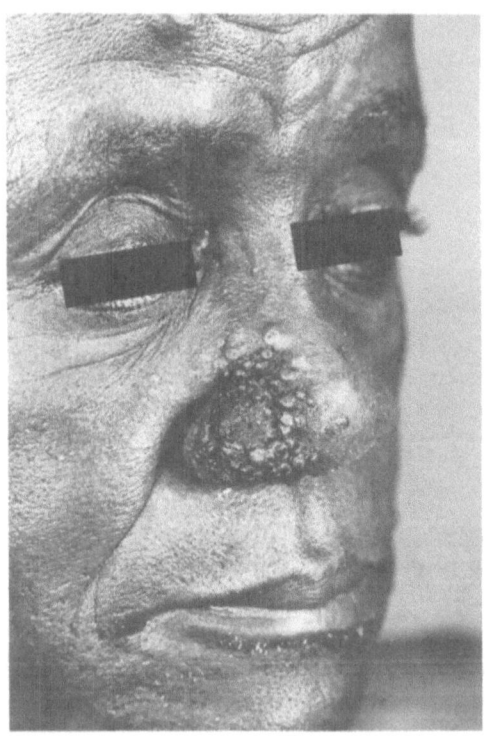

FIGURE 12-3 Crusting and ulceration on the nose of an Iranian man who had disseminated sporotrichosis. (Courtesy Homayoun Aram, M.D., Jerusalem, Israel.)

FIGURE 12-4 Crusting on the cheek of a Chinese boy. (Courtesy Institute of Dermatology, Chinese Academy of Medical Sciences, Jiangsu, People's Republic of China.)

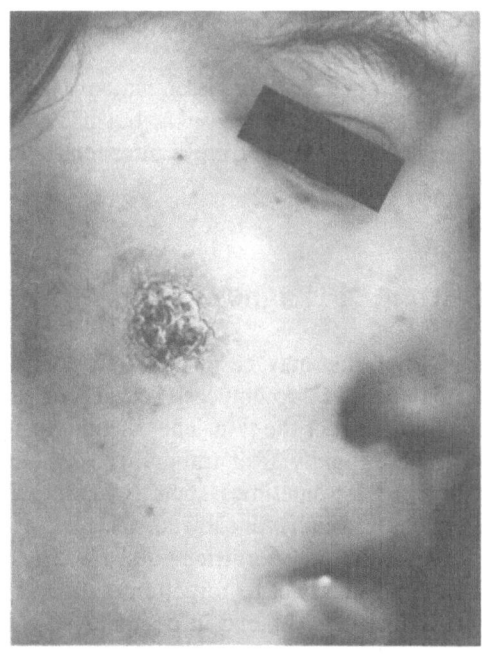

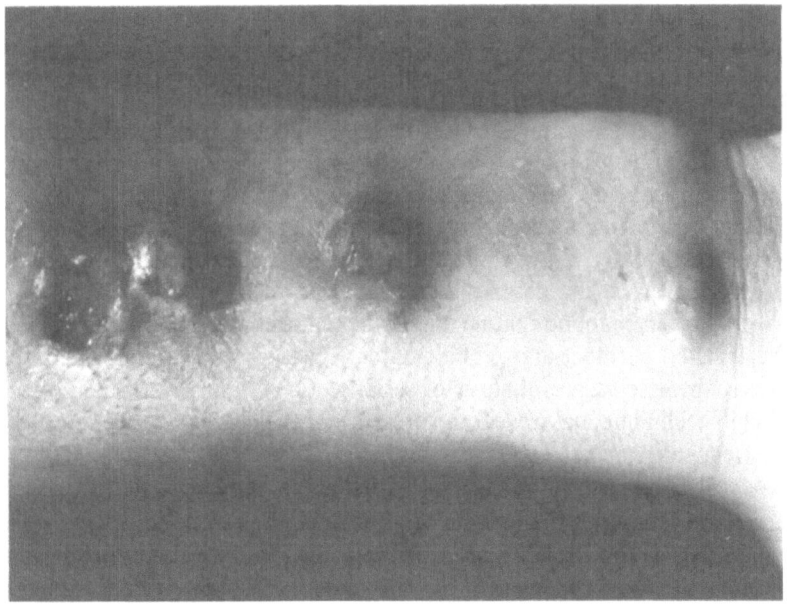

FIGURE 12-5   Draining ulcers on the arm. (Courtesy Institute of Dermatology, Chinese Academy of Medical Sciences, Jiangsu, People's Republic of China.)

erythematous nodules or pustules ascend the infected limb, ulcerating and discharging as they go.

Least common is the disseminated type of infection, which sometimes follows inhalation of *S. schenckii,* but is also reported to have arisen by direct systemic dissemination from a cutaneous lesion. In both instances, the outcome may be fatal.

Differential Diagnosis

The early lesion may be mistaken for many other diseases: North American blastomycosis, chromomycosis, cutaneous tuberculosis, or atypical mycobacterial infections of the skin. The essential feature is that sporotrichosis develops much more rapidly after trauma; thus, the disease can usually be recognized by its history. Sometimes, sporotrichosis can be confused with a pyoderma of recent onset, which will show all the signs of acute inflammation.

Frequently, the sporotrichoid chain of lesions will indicate the right diagnosis, but it must not be forgotten that other deep fungi, particularly chromomycosis, may also extend in a similar way, in which case laboratory investigations will be necessary to clarify the diagnosis.

Investigations

Usually, the most helpful method of investigation in a suspected case of sporotrichosis is to set up cultures from the ulcer exudate, although the fungus is not particularly plentiful in pus or affected tissue. If present, it will grow rapidly, producing a firm chocolate-brown colony.

Biopsies taken from a lesion will heal slowly, leaving considerable scarring, and should be avoided if the clinical diagnosis has been confirmed by positive culture. If, however, the diagnosis has not been recognized and a biopsy is taken, it wll often be found that no diagnostic features are demonstrable. There will be a mixed purulent and granulomatous reaction with numerous nonspecific microabscesses. Careful study of serial sections stained with the periodic acid-Schiff technique may reveal the presence of the *Sporotrix,* but such studies are frequently unsuccessful.

Rarely, it is possible to demonstrate an asteroid body, in which an eosinophilic stellate coating of the fungal cells known as the Splendore-Hoeppli phenomenon may be detected. This strange and unexplained abnormality is not diagnostic. It has been found in botryomycosis and various forms of phycomycosis.

Intradermal skin tests, complement fixation, and serum agglutination titers usually confuse clinicians more than they help them.

Treatment

The traditional method has been the use of a saturated solution of potassium iodide. The treatment schedule begins with 5 drops three times a day increasing by 1 drop per day per dose up to 30 or 40 drops daily, continued for four to six weeks or until symptoms of iodism supervene.

When allergy to potassium iodide exists, amphotericin B given intravenously is probably the best alternative treatment. Recent successful reports about ketoconazole 200 mg daily for three months suggest that this treatment is equally effective and easier to give.

Since the parasitic yeast phase of *S. schenckii* is very intolerant of heat above 37°C, smaller lesions have been found to respond well to hot compresses. An ingenious physician may wish to devise some method of applying warmth to larger areas.

Selected Readings

Dellatorre, DL, Lattanand, A, Buckley, HR, Urbach, F.: Fixed cutaneous sporotrichosis of the face. *J Am Acad Dermatol* 1982; 6:97.

Dolezal, JF: Blastomycoid sporotrichosis: Response to low-dose amphotericin. *J Am Acad Dermatol* 1981; 4:523.

Grekin, RH: Sporotrichosis: Two cases of exogenous second infection *J Am Acad Dermatol* 1984; 10:233.

Johnson, FB: Splendore-Hoeppli phenomenon, in Binford, CH, Connor, DH (eds), *Pathology of Tropical and Extraordinary Diseases*. Washington, DC, Armed Forces Institute of Pathology, 1976, vol 2, p 681.

Nusbaum, BP, Gulbas, N, Horwitz, N: Sporotrichosis acquired from a cat. *J Am Acad Dermatol* 1983; 8:386.

Read, SI, Sperling, LC: Feline sporotrichosis: Transmission to man. *Arch Dermatol* 1982; 118:429.

Smith, PW, Loomis, GW, Luckasen, JL, Osterholm, RK: Disseminated cutaneous sporotrichosis. *Arch Dermatol* 1981; 117:142.

Sperling, LC, Read, SI: Localized cutaneous sporotrichosis. *Int J Dermatol* 1983; 22:525.

Trejos, A, Ranirez, O: Local heat in the treatment of sporotrichosis. *Mycopathologia* 1966; 30:47.

Vanderveen, EE, Messenger, AL, Voorhees, JJ: Sporotrichosis in pregnancy. *Cutis* 1982; 30:761.

CHAPTER 13

Actinomycosis

As the nineteenth century progressed, workers in many parts of the world took an interest in discharging dermatological lesions that contained hard granules made of fungus. In 1877, friable yellow masses, now known as sulfur granules, were recognized in certain discharges; as they contained radiating filaments, the organisms were called ray fungi or actinomycetes. More recently, it has been realized that the actinomycetes are not true fungi but occupy a place between bacilli and the eumycetes.

Many types are now recognized: they include *Nocardia asteroides* and *Nocardia brasiliensis,* both of which are sometimes found to be the causative agent in certain cases of Madura foot (see chapter 11), while *N. asteroides* may also affect the lung and the brain, given the clinical picture of nocardiosis. Other forms of ray fungus have from time to time been isolated from skin lesions, the most important being *Actinomyces israelii,* an anaerobic organism that may live symbiotically in the mouth. Under certain conditions, it is responsible for the clinical condition known as actinomycosis.

This disease was first recognized in Europe, but is now rare in the more affluent countries. Most cases are found in developing countries, although here too the incidence seems to be decreasing. Men are afflicted more than women, and poor dental hygiene is a predisposing cause.

Etiology

A ray fungus *(Actinomyces bovis),* was originally isolated from lesions of the jaws of cattle, hence, the clinical term *lumpy jaw.* A few years later in 1878, James Israel found a similar organism in a similar lesion in a human being and appropriately named it *Actinomyces israelii.* There is some disagreement in the mycologic world as to whether these two are identical. (Mycologists have taken these organisms into their protective custody, making it necessary for authors to discuss actinomycosis among the fungus diseases!) Many names have been given variant actinomycetes isolated from the skin and the mouth. They all seem to be marginally different in the laboratory, but histopathologically they cannot be distinguished from *A. israelii.*

The basic difference between actinomycosis and mycetoma is that the latter is initiated by inoculation of aerobic organisms that can be found in nature as saprophytic flora of the soil. Actinomycosis, on the other hand, is caused by an anaerobic and endogenous actinomycete that affects internal organs before it spreads to the skin. Primary cutaneous actinomycosis is exceedingly rare.

It is not known how *A. israelii* spreads from person to person, and there is no scientific evidence to support the medical myth that the disease results from chewing straw or grasses.

Clinical Features

A. israelii, living as it does as a saprophyte in the mouth, seems to be able to invade the body in three sites and therefore shows three different clinical forms—on the face and neck, on the thorax, and on the abdominal wall.

Cervical-Facial Infections

These are probably caused by the actinomycete invading a periodontal abscess at the site of a carious tooth or dental extraction. It then spreads to the maxilla or the mandible, where periostitis and osteomyelitis develop. From there it extends through the subcutaneous tissue to the skin, where a pinkish-red nodule appears (Figure 13-1). Even in its earliest stages, this is recognizably adherent to deeper structures. The swelling slowly softens and fluctuates, becoming darker in color, and later breaks down to produce one or more sinuses from which discharges a serosanguinous pus containing the bright yellow granules giving the disease its name. At the same time, other nodules develop and coalesce, finally producing a board-hard induration traversed by numerous fistulae. The condition is usually painful, particularly during eating. If the disease spreads far enough, movements of the head and neck become limited. Brain abscesses even can develop.

Thoracic Actinomycosis

This is seen less frequently and invariably follows actinomycotic invasion of the lung. It probably cannot occur unless the lung tissue has previously been damaged by such diseases as tuberculosis or chronic bronchiectasis. Once established, however, it takes the usual course, with infection spreading outward,

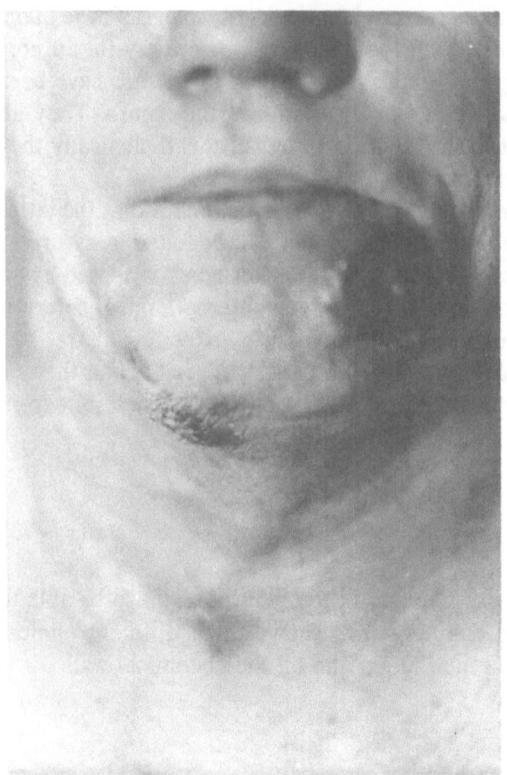

FIGURE 13-1 Lumpy jaw in a 40-year-old Philadelphia man.

involving first the ribs and then extending to the skin to produce an indurated area riddled with boggy nodules and discharging fistulae.

Abdominal Actinomycosis

This is the rarest of the three manifestations commonly cited. Somehow, the actinomycete, reaching the end of the small intestine, which it never seems to invade, establishes a slowly developing infection in the cecum or appendix. This then adheres to the abdominal wall, spreads through the musculature, and appears on the surface (usually in the lower right abdominal quadrant) as a boardlike induration. The diagnosis will be confirmable clinically only, when fistulae develop and allow the sulfur granules to surface.

Natural History

In all three of the classical manifestations the onset is insidious, and it takes many months or even years to produce a clinically recognizable picture.

Extension of infection is not necessarily directed outward (there is no evidence that the organism has an optimal temperature requirement), as it may spread to the orbit, the skull, or the brain from cervicofacial lesions, while in the abdomen direct extension to the liver, ovaries, kidney, and spine have all been known to complicate the disease.

If a secondary bacterial infection becomes established, a regional lymphadenitis may develop. Otherwise, lymph nodes are rarely affected other than by direct extension from a neighboring infection.

Until the advent of antibiotics, the condition was frequently fatal, and spontaneous resolution was not reported.

Differential Diagnosis

When the clinical picture is fully established, the diagnosis is incontrovertible, but in its early stages the disease may be confused with other chronic inflammations. In the absence of the diagnostic granules, a dental abscess or infected dental sinus may be suspected, but these are more acute and painful. Cutaneous tuberculosis (see Chapter 5) may be confusing early on, but it rarely leads to such a hard induration. Syphilitic gumma develops more rapidly and produces a punched-out ulcer, which looks quite different.

Malignant disease, amebic ulcers of the skin (see Chapter 21), and sporotrichosis (see Chapter 12) have all to be considered. Mycetoma can usually be differentiated by the history of the infection starting superficially and penetrating deeper as time goes on.

Detailed laboratory studies will be needed to separate actinomycosis from botryomycosis (see Chapter 14).

Investigations

The diagnosis stands or falls on the demonstration of friable sulfur granules that differ from those of a mycetoma, which are harder and usually of different colors. *N. asteroides, N. brasiliensis, Streptomyces madurae,* and *Cephalosporium falciforme* are the most difficult to distinguish. They all have yellowish-white granules, but the *A. israelli* is a brighter sulfur yellow.

Attempts should always be made to culture the granules in a brain-heart infusion agar. A rough, dry, creamy-white colony will grow anaerobically, showing fine filaments and bacillary elements that are Gram positive and not acid resistant.

Histologically, a biopsy from an actinomycotic lesion will show the granules, stained purple by hematoxylin and eosin, enveloped by a purulent exudate in the middle of necrotic tissue. Occasionally, an actinomycotic granule is found living saprophytically in a crypt of a tonsil that has been removed for a different reason. In such cases, it will not be surrounded by an adherent pustular exudate.

Treatment

A. israelii is not a fungus and responds well to most antibiotics—it is rarely
necessary to use anything except penicillin. The dosage must be high, usually
four to five million units intramuscularly every day for at least a year. When
not feasible, similar high doses of oral penicillin may be used. Although this
may successfully eradicate the infection, the subsequent mess of puckered and
scarred tissue is best avoided by widespread excision of the lesion shortly after
the onset of penicillin therapy. When the patient is allergic to penicillin or the
drug is not available, broad-spectrum antibiotics such as tetracycline or erythromycin 250 mg four times a day can be used. Underlying deformities of bone
or spread of infection to abdominal organs may provide a stern challenge to
stern challenge to even the most inventive surgeon. Fortunately, this is less and
less necessary as the twentieth century wears on. It is possible that the decreasing incidence of actinomycosis may be the result of widespread use of antibiotics, which kill the saprophyte before it has a chance to become a pathogen.

Follow-up

Patients who have been treated may relapse if any organisms have managed
to take shelter in a nest of necrotic scar tissue. Any suggestion of recurrence
should be treated with a different antibiotic in high doses for a minimum of
three months.

Selected Readings

Binford, CH, Dooley, JR: Actinomycosis, in Binford, CH, Connor, DA (eds): *Pathol-
    ogy of Tropical and Extraordinary Diseases*. Washington, DC, Armed Forces
    Institute of Pathology, 1976, pp 552–554.
Israel, J: Neue Beobachtungen auf dem Gebiete der Mykosen des Menchen. *Virchows
    Arch [Pathol Anat]* 1878; 74:15.
Kosh, G, Lalitha, MK, Samraj, T, Mathai, KV: Brain abscess and other protean man-
    ifestations of actinomycosis. *Am J Trop Med Hyg* 1981; 30:139.
Peabody, JW, Seabury, JA: Actinomycosis and nocardiosis. *Am J Med* 1960; 28:99.
Robbins, TS, Scott, SA: Actinomycosis—the disease and its treatment. *Drug Int Clin
    Pharm* 1981; 15:99.

CHAPTER 14

Botryomycosis

There is considerable confusion about the origins of the dermatosis known as botryomycosis. Some say it was first described by Bollinger in 1870 as a disease of horses' lungs, while others claim it was originally recognized by veterinary surgeons as a fungating granuloma found in horses as a complication of castration. In either case, the name was not used until many years after Bollinger's description: it was coined because granules seen in the pus somewhat resembled a bunch of grapes. To add to the confusion, Radcliffe Crocker used the same name to describe what is now known as granuloma pyogenicum, but this cherry-red tumor has nothing to do with the condition nowadays called botryomycosis.

Botryomycosis occurs anywhere in the world. The word is a complete misnomer as the disease it has come to describe is bacterial in origin and not related in any way to the eumycetes or the actinomycetes. It is discussed here because of its clinical similarities with actinomycosis, Madura foot, and the other mycetomas.

Etiology

This chronic suppurative process is caused by organisms that clump together in the tissue to form granules. A number of different bacteria have been isolated—*Staphylococcus pyogenes*, *Staphylococcus aureus*, and *Pseudomonas aeruginosa* being most commonly reported. It is not certain what causes these common organisms to behave in such an atypical way, but there may be a factor (perhaps antistreptolysin O) inhibiting normal neutrophil chemotaxis. Patients often have associated systemic disease—diabetes, active hepatitis, cystic fibrosis, follicular mucinosis, or gross malnutrition.

Clinical Features

The condition is recognizable only when it occurs in the skin. A similar pathologic process in internal organs cannot be diagnosed clinically. A group of inflammatory nodules appears, becomes larger and proliferates, and then forms abscesses from which draining sinuses will discharge soft yellow granules. These lesions may be embedded in a painful inflammatory edema, but the swelling is usually not extensive (Figure 14-1).

It is not confined to any part of the skin, although a mild predilection for the hands and feet suggests that traumatic inoculation could play a part in the causation of the disease. In cases where only the skin is infected, the prognosis is good, as the lesion may regress; however, in patients with associated systemic disease, spontaneous cure is less likely.

Differential Diagnosis

The condition can easily be confused with other diseases from which colored granules are found in pus discharging from deep sinuses in the skin. In Madura foot and the other so-called mycetomas, the causative agents are true fungi or anaerobic actinomycetes, and their granules are exceedingly hard. Actinomy-

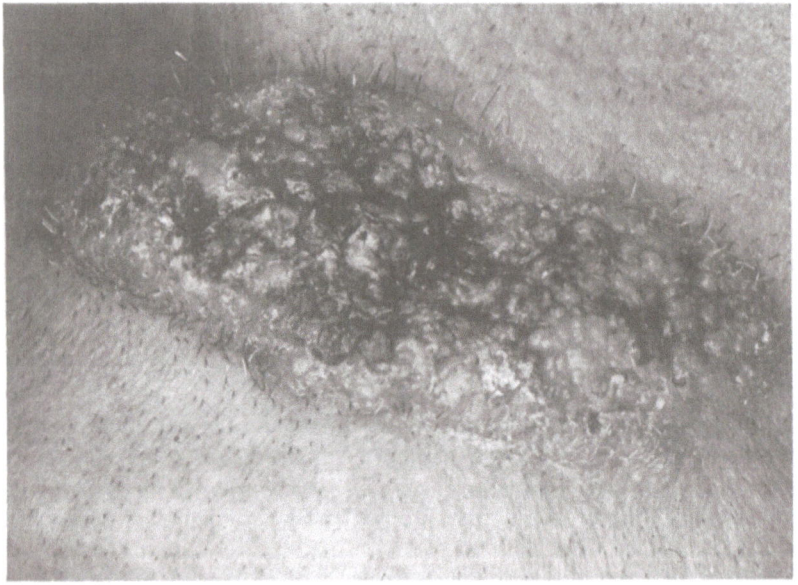

FIGURE 14-1   Heaped-up granulating tissue that is quite friable.

cosis, caused by an anaerobic organism that is neither a fungus or a bacterium, produces bright sulfur-yellow granules, which are more friable than those seen in the true mycetomas. In botryomycosis, the grapelike granules are softer and a paler yellow. Other helpful features are that it rarely affects the actinomycosis sites and does not show a board-hard induration.

Investigations

Although it is sometimes necessary to repeat the search on several occasions, granules will ultimately be found that consist of large clusters of bacteria, coated by an amorphous eosinophilic material. When cultured, these granules will reveal diagnosable features.

Histopathologic section will usually show granules to be surrounded by pus and necrosis; sometimes a liquifying tuberculoid granuloma has caused a mistaken diagnosis of sporotrichosis.

In view of the suggestion that there is an associated deficiency of leukocyte chemotaxis, suitable investigations should be carried out if laboratory facilities are available.

Treatment

A satisfactory response to antibiotics is to be expected provided the causative organism is suitably susceptible, and the patient's progress is not complicated by systemic abnormalities. Without benefit of bacterial cultures, penicillin G three to four million units daily for several months will usually induce satisfactory recovery. Some cases have been reported in which penicillin was ineffective; this was probably due to bacterial resistance rather than to some complicated immunologic feature of the disease. In such cases, other antibiotics should be used, such as synthetic penicillins (cloxacillin 500 mg), erythromycin 250 mg, or tetracycline 250 mg all four times a day.

As in actinomycosis, it may be necessary to seek surgical assistance to obtain the best cosmetic result.

Selected Readings

Bishop, GF, Greer, KE, Horwitz, DA: Pseudomonas botryomycosis. *Arch Dermatol* 1976; 112:1568.

Bollinger, O: Mycosis der Lunge Bein Pferde. *Virchows Arch [Pathol Anat]* 1870; 49:583.

Brunken, RC, Lichon-Chao, N, van den Broek, H: Immunologic abnormalities in botryomycosis. *J Am Acad Dermatol* 1983; 9:428.

Harman, RRM, English, MP, Halford, M, Saihan, EM, Greenham, LW: Botryomycosis: A complication of extensive follicular mucinosis. *Br J Dermatol* 1980;
102:215.

Leibowitz, R, Asvat, MS, Kalla, AA, Wing, G: Extensive botryomycosis in a patient
with diabetes and chronic active hepatitis. *Arch Dermatol* 1981; 117:739.

Picou, A, Batres, E, Jarratt, M: Botryomycosis: A bacterial cause of mycetoma. *Arch
Dermatol* 1979; 115:609.

Chapter 15

Rhinosporidiosis

Rhinosporidiosis, first recognized in Buenos Aires, Argentina, is caused by an organism that was originally detected by Seeber in 1896. He thought he had found a new protozoan organism but it is now believed that the causative agent is a fungus, probably a member of the phycomycetes, and it has been named *Rhinosporidium seeberi*. The disease is endemic in south India and Sri Lanka and has been seen sporadically in most countries, from the United States to Malaysia and from Argentina to Poland. It may occur at any age and is more commonly diagnosed in men than in women in a ratio of 10 to 1.

Etiology

The method of transmission is unknown; some authorities believe that stagnant water is the chief source of infection, while others believe it is transmitted by infected dust. A similar condition has been found in cattle and horses, but transmission to laboratory animals has not been convincing.

The infecting spore is a small, round body approximately 6 to 7 μ in diameter, with a well-defined limiting membrane, a nucleus, and a karyosome. It increases in size as repeated nuclear divisions take place. By the time it has reached 100 μ in diameter, a thick cellulose layer is deposited on the inner aspect of the surrounding chitinous membrane: on one point of this a thinning occurs to form a pore. Further nuclear divisions produce a sporangium ultimately containing several thousand spores. The sporangia are white and are often 300 μ in diameter, just visible to the naked eye. Ultimately spores are liberated by rupture of the sporangium at the pore.

Clinical Features

As the name suggests, this fungus primarily affects the nose and nasopharynx. A chronic granulomatous reaction produces pedunculated polyps that soon interfere with breathing. They are friable and bleed easily, the epistaxis often being combined with a mucinous discharge. When viewed closely, the larger of the white sporangia are seen scattered in the erythematous polyp, producing what has been called a strawberrylike lesion (a simile more accurate than most) (Figure 15-1).

The condition is included in this book because lesions are not necessarily confined to the nose; they have also been seen on the conjunctivae, mouth, lips, ears, scalp, penis, vagina, and rectum, where they start as papillomatous or subcutaneous nodules, frequently pruritic, which later become warty and exude a mucinous material in which sporangia can be detected with the aid of a hand lens.

If the conjunctiva is affected, there is initial lacrimation and photophobia succeeded by the development of different-shaped growths, the lesions being sessile when growing from the bulbar conjunctiva and pedunculated on the palpebral conjunctiva.

On the genitalia, they may be mistaken for condyloma latum if the sporangia are not recognized.

Natural History

Epistaxis and nasal blockage are the main early symptoms. Slowly the nasal cavity becomes full of granulomatous polyps that may reach an enormous size, spilling out into pharynx and protruding through the nostrils to hang over the upper lip. Occasionally, it has been reported that the disease has regressed within a few weeks of onset, but other cases are known to have lasted more than 30 years. Recurrence is likely, even in cases that appear to be doing well, so it is unwise ever to tell patients that they are completely cured. Rhinosporidiosis is rarely fatal, although deaths have been reported following generalized dissemination of the disease and also from direct obstruction of the trachea and bronchus.

Differential Diagnosis

In the nose or mouth, the strawberrylike lesions will establish the diagnosis easily and separate it from the many other conditions that may develop nasal polyps.

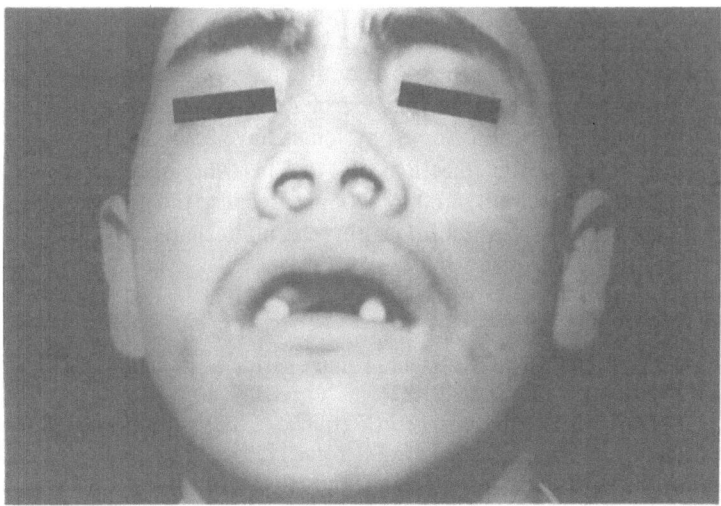

FIGURE 15-1   Strawberrylike lesions in the nares. (Courtesy Arturo Tapia, M.D., Panama City, Panama.)

When it is fully established, the classical hypertrophy and sclerosis of rhinoscleroma (see Chapter 16) should not cause too much diagnostic confusion. Patients with paracoccidioidomycosis, yaws, tertiary syphilis, leishmaniasis, and lepromatous leprosy may all complain of epistaxis or nasal blockage, but other signs will usually be visible on the skin.

Investigations

An impression smear from the surface of a polyp mixed with a drop of water and examined under the microscope will probably reveal characteristic sporangia, while the periodic acid-Schiff stain clearly demonstrates the inner portion of the wall, which tends to be birefringent. Nasal discharge may be studied in the same way or with Romanovsky's stain. Rhinosporidial sporangia differ from coccidioidomycosis sporangia, which are smaller (up to 80 μ in diameter) and contain much smaller spores (about 2.5 μ).

Biopsy of one of the polyps, stained routinely with hematoxylin and eosin, will show sporangia in all stages of development. They are sometimes surrounded by acute inflammation resulting from release of spores into the tissue, but more commonly a chronic granulomatous reaction is seen with epithelioid cells and Langhans' cells. As will be expected of such bright red lesions, vascular dilation is a conspicuous histologic feature.

Treatment

There is no known chemotherapeutic or antifungal agent. The only treatment that can be recommended is the removal of lesions by excision or curettage followed by electrodesiccation. Some physicians have helped patients by treating them with intramuscular injections of 2 to 5 percent aqueous tartar emetic or ethylstilbamidine to a total of 60 to 120 mg. Because the disease is not fatal and may abate on its own, watchful waiting is an alternative therapy.

Selected Readings

Allen RFWK, Dave, ML: The treatment of rhinosporidiosis in man based on a study of cases. *Indian Med Gaz* 1946; 71:376.

Ashworth, JH: On *rhinsporidium seeberi* (Wernicke, 1903) with special reference to its sporulation and affinities. *Trans R Soc Edin* 1923; 53:46.

Chitravel, V, Subramanian, S, Sundaram, BM, et al: Rhinosporidiosis in a South Indian village. *Sabouraudia* 1980; 18:241.

Kannan Kutty, N, Prabakharan, N, Monsurate, J: Oculosporidiosis. *Far East Med J* 1968; 4:118.

Ramanathan, K, Ahmad, U, Kutty, M, et al: Rhinosporidiosis in Malaysia. *Med J Malaya* 1968; 22:276.

CHAPTER 16

Rhinoscleroma

There is evidence that rhinoscleroma, sometimes simply called scleroma, was known to the Amerindians of pre-Colombian America. The definitive descriptions were made by Hebra and Kaposi (Kohn) in the 1870s, at which time endemic areas were found in Galesia, other parts of the Austro-Hungarian Empire, and Russia. In more recent times, cases have been reported in China, Egypt, Israel, Iraq, Indonesia, and North America. At present, the highest incidence seems to be in Venezuela and parts of Central America. Sporadic cases of this multilating disease probably may be found in any part of the world.

Etiology

Although Koch's postulates are not entirely fulfilled, since the disease has never been produced experimentally, most authorities believe that *Klebsiella rhinoscleromatis* is the causative organism. It is a Gram-negative, encapsulated bacillus that is found singly or in short chains.

There is very little evidence that the disease is contagious; occasionally, two or three cases are seen in a family, but most patients have no such background. It is possible that climatic or environmental conditions or immunologic incompetence play a part in the development of the disease. The incubation period may be very long. If so, confirmatory history of contact may be difficult to obtain.

Clinical Features

When the condition is fully established, there is extensive hyperplasia of the nose and the center of the face. It is an alarming sight. A chronic inflammatory reaction invades the floor of the nose (Figure 16-1) and the nasal septum and

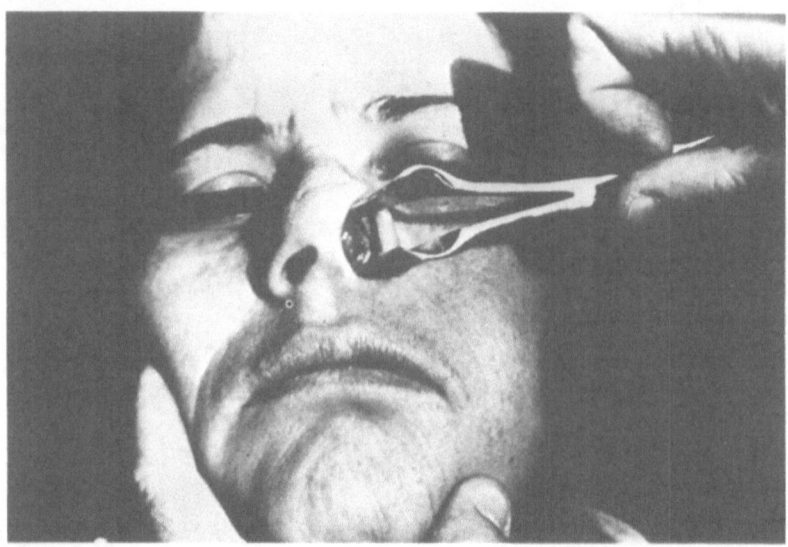

FIGURE 16-1   Early lesions in the nose showing tumorous overgrowth. (Courtesy Francisco Kerdel-Vegas, M.D., Jacinto Convit, M.D., Bernard Gordon, M.D., and Mauricio Goihman-Yahr, M.D., Caracas, Venezuela.)

extends outward to the nose and upper lip, downward through the palate, backward to the larynx, or up to the orbit. This massive tumorous overgrowth hinders breathing to such an extent that patients may only be able to breath through the mouth, while palatal involvement will modify the resonance of speech.

Occasionally, the condition remains untreated for years, and slowly the infective element is replaced by the fibrosis that caused it to be called rhinoscleroma; this may involve the larynx and even the bronchi (Figure 16-2).

Natural History

The whole process of development is prolonged, taking many years after the appearance of the earliest symptoms. The first stage is a rhinitic infection, when what seems to be a comon cold becomes more than usually intense, with headache, respiratory distress, and foul-smelling nasal discharge. The mucous membranes of the nose become hypertrophied and later atrophy. These changes are first seen at the base of the nasal cavity. The granulations creep up the nasal septum and the sides of the nose, slowly obstructing the nasal cavity. At this stage, the coryzal symptoms disappear, thickening of the tissues increases, and infiltration steadily produces the nodular and hypertrophic condition that is typical of the established infection. As time goes on, the soft, boggy granulomatous tissue hardens, leaving the unfortunate patient with a

FIGURE 16-2 Late lesions showing extensive fibrosis of nose and lips. (Courtesy Mohsen Soliman, M.D., Cairo, Egypt.)

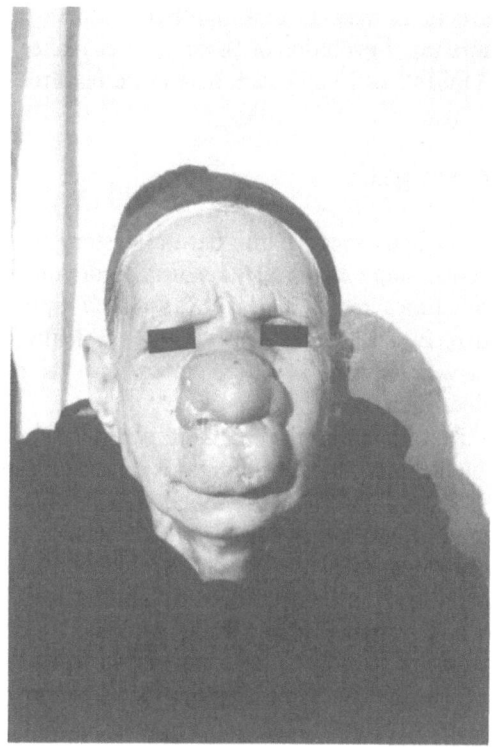

blocked nose, extensively involved central portions of the face, and a sclerosis spreading into the larynx and bronchi.

Differential Diagnosis

Although many chronic bacterial diseases affect the nose and center of the face, most of them tend to leave atrophy rather than hypertrophy. Tuberculosis, yaws, tertiary syphilis, and lepromatous leprosy may all be suspected in the earlier stages of rhinoscleroma, but when the classical hypertrophy (sometimes known as Hebra's nose) is fully established, the diagnosis should not be in doubt.

Certain of the deep mycoses, especially paracoccidioidomycosis, may produce hypertrophic granulations that bleed easily, and rhinosporidiosis (see Chapter 15) causes a granuloma that is much softer and studded with clearly visible sporangiophores.

Several malignant conditions may cause confusion: midline facial granuloma, Wegener's granulomatosis, the lymphomata, and even squamous cell carcinoma may all look like hypertrophic tumors blocking the nose, but the more rapid evolution of these diseases makes it unlikely that the diagnosis will be mistaken. In all cases, diagnostic features can be seen histologically.

Investigations

Throughout most of the natural history of rhinoscleroma, from the earliest rhinitic stage onward, the causative organism can be demonstrated in tissue. Sometimes known as the encapsulated diplococcus of Frisch, it is Gram negative, 2 to 3 μ long, and grows aerobically on blood agar. *Klebsiella rhinoscleromatis* may be differentiated from the other *Klebsiellae,* as it is lethal to mice.

The diagnosis may be more certainly confirmed by the histologic picture, which shows, in addition to an extensive plasma-cell infiltrate associated with the Russell colloid bodies found in any infiltrate containing many plasma cells, numerous Mikulicz' cells, whose presence is diagnostic. There are large, round, vacuolated histiocytes, often more than 100 μ in diameter. They have eccentric nuclei, and despite their foamy appearance, they do not contain lipid. If the section is stained with a bacterial stain, the Frisch's bacilli will be seen in the cytoplasm. Mikulicz' cells increase in number as the disease progresses.

Serologic reactions ranging from complement fixation to agglutination tests are not helpful, and attempts to provoke a cutaneous reaction from suspensions of the Frisch's bacillus have been indifferently successful.

Treatment

Rhinoscleroma does not respond well to penicillin or the sulfa drugs, but chloramphenicol and tetracycline have both been found helpful if used in large doses for a long period. Streptomycin is probably the drug of choice and should be given 1 g daily for at least three months.

As the disease resolves, there may be considerable residual deformity, and surgical assistance may be needed to reduce the nasal obstruction or cosmetic damage.

Selected Readings

Goldman, L: Pre-Columbian rhinoscleroma. *Arch Dermatol* 1979; 115:106.

Kerdel-Vegas, F, Convit, J, Gordon, B, et al: *Rhinoscleroma.* Springfield, Ill, Charles C Thomas, 1963.

Miller, RH, et al: *Klebsiella rhinoscleromatis:* A clinical and pathogenic otolaryngeal enigma. *Head Neck Surg* 1979; 87:212.

CHAPTER 17

North American Blastomycosis

The deep fungal condition was first recognized in North America. In the early stages of the disease, the nondescript collection of signs and symptoms is often misdiagnosed; in fact, when the first known patient was seen in Philadelphia in the early 1890s the diagnosis was missed. Not until later, in Baltimore, did Caspar Gilchrist notice the yeast bodies in a histopathologic specimen and define the disease that sometimes has been called Gilchrist's disease.

Originally found only in North America, particularly along the valleys of the Mississippi, Missouri, and Ohio rivers, the disease seems to be extending southward and is being recognized more frequently in Mexico, Central America, and even in South America. Sporadic cases have also been detected in the Middle East and all parts of Africa from Tunisia to South Africa. It is particularly prevalent in Zimbabwe.

Etiology

Blastomyces dermatitidis is a dimorphic fungus that grows easily on Sabouraud's agar. It is not known how the disease is transmitted, and there is no evidence that it is contagious. There are a few reports of isolation of the organism from soil, an important finding, as most patients are men, and more than three-quarters of them are exposed to soil in their work. An astonishingly high percentage of patients are over 40 years of age. A few pathologists have acquired the disease by direct cutaneous inoculation, but such cases are extremely rare and clinically atypical in that they show a strong tendency to spontaneous recovery.

Clinical Features

Apart from the few cases of direct inoculation, it is believed that in most cases North American blastomycosis afflicts the skin following infection of the lung. Starting as a small papule or pustule (or, very rarely, a vesicle), the lesion, which may be single or multiple, enlarges to form nodules that ulcerate and discharge pus. The center of the lesion heals, leaving a paper-thin layer of skin, while crusting and scaling extend peripherally to produce verruciform lesions interspersed with pustules. As the years go by, the patch extends slowly, leaving extensively atrophic scarring, ringed with active warty granulomatous lesions. If the eyelids are affected, an ectropion may occur; mucous membranes are only rarely involved (Figures 17-1, 17-2).

Single lesions occur on the limbs or face, but if multiple infection occurs, the areas are frequently symmetrical and usually on the trunk.

At the same time, the disease may spread to subcutaneous tissue and extend to the bones and joints, the resulting osteomyelitis producing draining sinuses of the skin. The central nervous system or the renal tract can be affected also. Such widely disseminated disease usually has a poor prognosis, even if the cause is recognized and suitable treatment instituted.

Natural History

Pulmonary blastomycosis precedes the appearance of cutaneous lesions in almost all cases. It is suspected that this is due to the inhalation of spores from the soil, leading to a respiratory infection that may be symptom-free but more

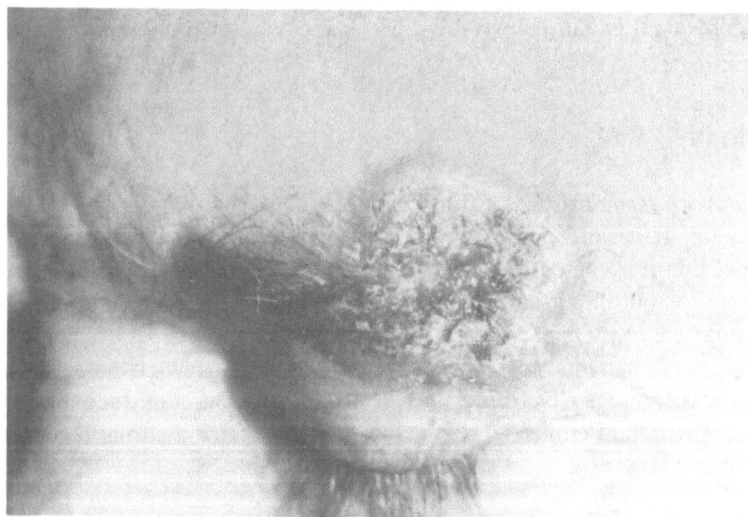

FIGURE 17-1   Crust lesion with sharp border extending from the eyebrow.

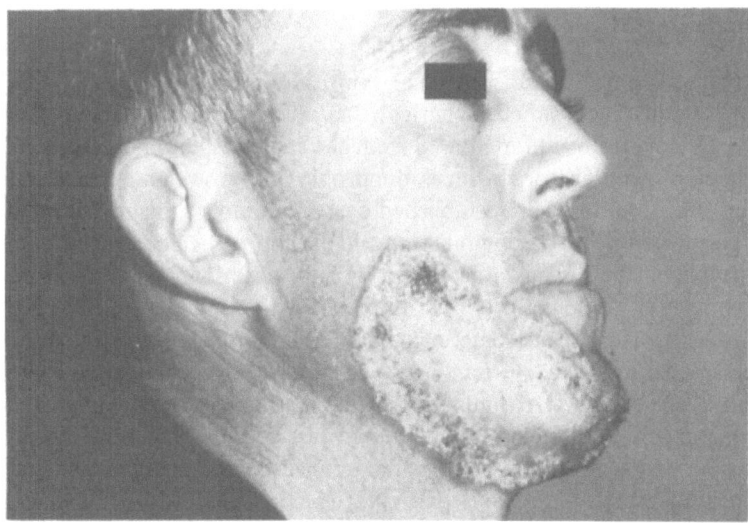

FIGURE 17-2 Crusted lesion with sharp border; some atrophy may already be perceived.

usually mimics pulmonary tuberculosis, with hemoptysis, dyspnea, loss of weight, low-grade fever, and sometimes even erythema nodosum. This picture draws attention to the lungs, and radiographic examination usually shows widespread miliary lesions but rarely cavitation.

Dissemination of infection to the skin may be delayed for a very long period; a recent case with multiple skin lesions had an episode of "pneumonia" 50 years previously, when he was working in an endemic area. It is postulated that with age an impaired immunologic activity can permit a flare-up and dissemination of an infection that has been dormant in the lung for many years. This theory would explain the late age of onset in such a high percentage of cases.

A less common means of infection is through primary inoculation. Animals, including horses, dogs, and cats, are known to have had the disease: in a recorded case, localized blastomycosis developed after a dog bite. In such cases, the incubation period is only a matter of months, and such lesions do not usually spread.

Differential Diagnosis

Clinically, the scarring granulomas may be mistaken for tuberculosis, syphilis, pyoderma gangrenosum, or bromoderma, as well as for other deep fungus infections. The clinical picture alone is rarely diagnostic. Paracoccidioidomycosis (see chapter 18) usually affects the mouth or nasal cavity, which is rarely the case in the North American variety of blastomycosis.

Investigations

Microscopic examination of pus or of skin scrapings may show *Blastomyces dermatitidis* as thick-walled, spherical, budding yeast cells (about 10 μ in diamter). They can be differentiated from the spores of chromomycosis, which are golden-brown. The organism is dimorphic and grows as a yeast at body temperature. If cultures are established on Sabouraud's agar at room temperature, a mycelial phase predominates in which short pedicules attach the spores to the hyphae. The organism grows slowly and takes four to six weeks before dirty-white, fluffy colonies are fully established. The spores can be seen fairly easily in histologic section, sometimes lying freely in the tissue, but more often are recognized living in the Langhan's giant cells. If special stains have not been used, the spores give a punched-out appearance to the cytoplasm. With the periodic acid-Schiff stain, the budding yeast cells can be clearly seen.

As the clinical diagnosis often remains unsuspected and pus may not be examined for spores, biopsy is of particular value in establishing the diagnosis. A typical lesion will show epithelial hyperplasia and acanthosis overlying extensive tuberculoid granulation tissue, which is mixed with numerous microabscesses. An unusually high number of Langhan's giant cells may cause the disease to be suspected, particularly if they have the punched-out appearance produced by unstained intracellular spores. In paracoccidioidomycosis, the spores are much larger (30 μ) and show multiple budding.

If a patient is suspected of having North American blastomycosis, the chest should be x-rayed, and the pulmonary lesions that are almost invariably present will have to be differentiated from tuberculosis or sarcoidosis by examination of the sputum, use of the tuberculin test, or even bronchoscopy.

Serologic tests, including complement fixation and immunodiffusion, are frequently not sensitive or specific enough. Often there is considerable antigenic overlap with *Histoplasma capsulatum* and *Coccidioides immitis*. The blastomycin skin test is useful only for epidemiologic purposes.

Treatment

Potassium iodide was formerly used to treat this disease. Later, this was replaced by 2-hydroxystilbamidine, but many patients relapsed. Amphotericin B given in standard doses up to 2 g has been more effective, but currently, ketoconazole 400 mg orally each day for several weeks has been shown to be curative and is recommended.

It is unwise to treat cases of cutaneous North American blastomycosis without careful watch for deeper infections. Regular chest x-rays should be taken to observe the progress of any concomitant pulmonary activity. The deeper infection may still need treatment after the skin lesions have resolved. There is a percentage of fatality with all known methods of therapy, and sometimes it is necessary to use more than one medication.

Selected Readings

Hashimoto, K, Kaplan, RJ, Daman, LA, et al: Pustular blastomycosis. *Int J Dermatol* 1977; 16:277.

Henchy, FP, Daniel, CR, Omura, EF, Kheir, SM: North American blastomycosis: An unusual clinical manifestation. *Arch Dermatol* 1982; 118:287.

Hudson, CP, Callen, JP: Systemic blastomycosis treated with ketonconazole. *Arch Dermatol* 1984; 120:536.

Logsdon, MT, Jones, HE: North American blastomycosis: A review. *Cutis* 1979; 24:524.

McClune, MA, Rogers, RS, Roberts, DG: Laryngeal presentation of blastomycosis. *Int J Dermatol* 1980; 19:263.

Sweeney, EW, Franks, A, Silva-Hunter, M: An unusual case of North American blastomycosis in New Jersey. *Cutis* 1982; 30:199.

CHAPTER 18

Paracoccidioidomycosis

To avoid confusion with North American blastomycosis, it is better that this disease, which has in the past been called South American or Brazilian blastomycosis, should be known as paracoccidioidomycosis. The disease extends from Mexico to Chile, with its highest incidence in the state of São Paolo in Brazil. It has probably never been acquired naturally outside this area.

Etiology

As with many of the deep fungus infections, the causative organism, *Paracoccidioides braziliensis,* is found in the soil; consequently, agricultural workers are frequently affected. The fact that almost all cases start in the mouth has stimulated the suggestion that the disease may be acquired as the result of cleaning teeth with fragments of wood, but this would not explain the greater incidence in men (90 percent of all cases).

Clinical Features

The typical lesion of paracoccidioidomycosis is seen in a middle-aged man, 45 to 50 years old, who has a very painful granulomatous condition of the buccal and/or nasal mucosa (Figure 18-1). An ulcerative stomatitis spreads across the mouth to the tonsils, and laryngeal and pulmonary lesions are also found. Authorities disagree as to whether the pulmonary or the oral-nasal lesions are the first to develop. The ulcerated tissue proliferates to form hyperemic edematous granulations known as mulberry erosions (Figure 18-2) (a mulberry is

FIGURE 18-1 Painful granulomatous crusted lesions on a
Brazilan man. (Courtesy Sebastião Sampaio, M.D., São
Paulo, Brazil.)

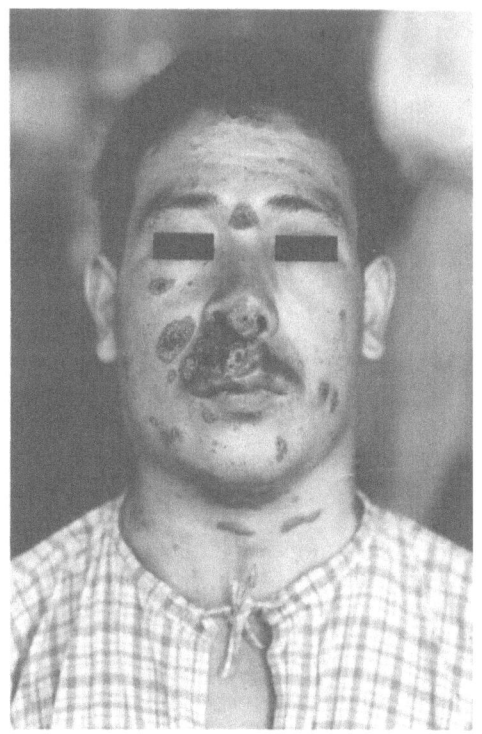

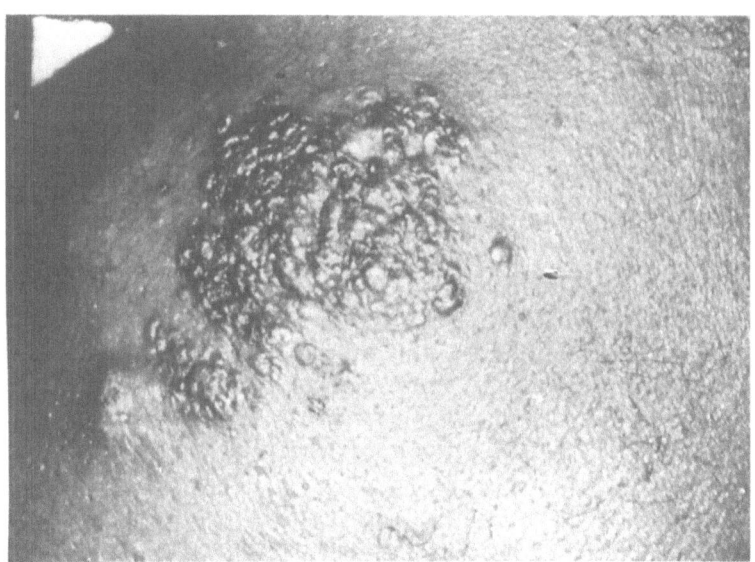

FIGURE 18-2   Mulberry type of granulation tissue.

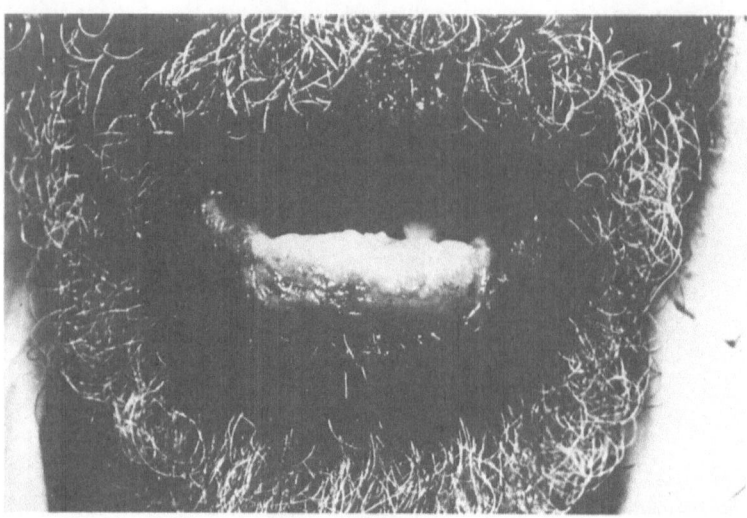

FIGURE 18-3   Erosion of the lips and destruction of the gums resulting in loss of teeth. (Courtesy Jacinto Convit, M.D., and Mauricio Goihman-Yahr, M.D., Caracas, Venezuela.)

a purple fruit resembling a raspberry), which can be found in the nose, on the palate, the gums (where as a consequence the teeth frequently fall out) (Figure 18-3), the tongue (Figure 18-4), the tonsils, and the larynx.

At the same time, ulcerated and crusting granulomata may spread to the skin of the mouth and around the nostrils, and the cervical lymph nodes enlarge to form an adherent suppurating mass clinically indistinguishable from a tuberculous adenitis or scrofuloderma.

Natural History

The incubation period is probably from five to ten years. As a result, the disease is almost completely unknown in children. Spontaneous regression of the condition has not been reported, but many patients seem to have some resistance. As the infection extends slowly, a degree of delayed hypersensitivity (type iv) can be shown by suitable skin tests. Less fortunate individuals are anergic, and the disease not only spreads locally but extends systemically throughout the body.

In such cases, the lungs and spleen are invariably involved, and lesions are also seen in the intestines and the liver, while the adrenals, the bones, and the central nervous system do not escape. About 50 percent of untreated patients have a slowly progressive fatal disease; the patient may die of peritonitis, meningitis, or even cachexia resulting from the painful oral lesions.

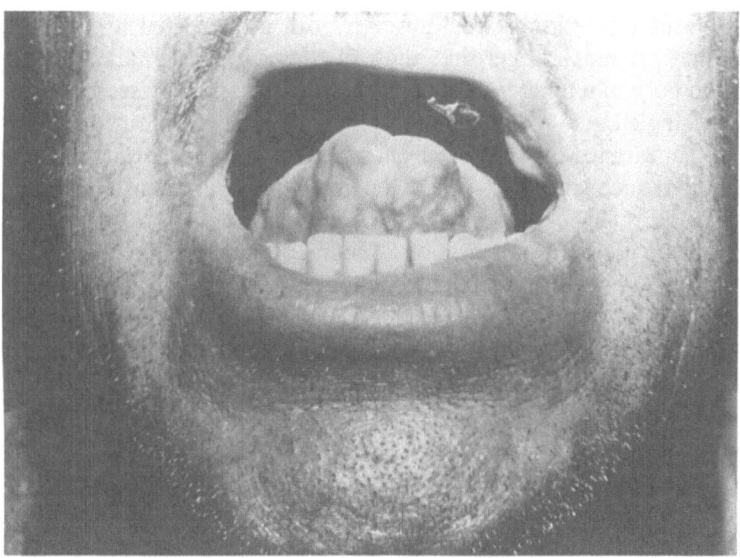

FIGURE 18-4   Proliferation of granulomatous tissue on the tongue. (Courtesy Sebastião Sampaio, M.D., São Paulo, Brazil.)

Differential Diagnosis

There should be no trouble in differentiating paracoccidioidomycosis from North American blastomycosis. The latter has a marked tendency to atrophy, which is not found in the South American disease, while *P. braziliensis* affects the mouth, the spleen, and the alimentary tract, three areas rarely if ever troubled by North American blastomycosis.

It is often difficult to determine whether the lung lesions are caused by paracoccidioidomycosis or tuberculosis. Hypertrophic conditions of the nose (rhinosporidiosis, rhinosceroma, or some cases of fungating squamous cell carcinoma) do not cause the teeth to fall out, nor are they usually associated with a suppurating cervical adenitis. Actinomycosis, especially if it invades the upper jaw, may sometimes mimic paracoccidioidomycosis, but the brawny swelling and the bright yellow granules should clarify matters. The American form of mucocutaneous leishmaniasis may also be suspected in the early stages; it does not, however, spread to the lungs or the abdominal organs.

Investigations

P. braziliensis is another of the diphasic organisms that appear as budding yeast cells at body temperature and produce mycelia when cultured at room temperature. Examination of fresh tissue or of discharge from the mulberry lesions or pus from the cervical abscesses can be expected to show typical spores. They are much larger than those of *Blastomyces dermatitidis*, ranging from 30 to 60 μ in diameter. Although they are occasionally seen to be reproducing by single budding, much more frequently many buds surround the cell, giving an appearance that has been compared to a ship's wheel. It must not be forgotten that such large cells when seen in a biopsy will themselves have been sectioned, and the whole spore will not be present.

Attempts to grow the organism on Sabouraud's agar will produce the mycelial form. If it is cultured on blood agar at 37°C, the yeast form will predominate.

Histologic section will show an epithelioid granuloma mixed with a polymorphonuclear infiltration, similar to the histology of North American blastomycosis, but here the causative organism is much larger and only rarely intracellular.

An intradermal skin test with paracoccidiodin will produce a reaction in 48 hours if the patient has any innate resistance to infection. As in leprosy, the test will be negative in anergic patents with the disseminated form of infection. There is a complement-fixation test that gives rising titers as the infection spreads. This investigation, combined with a precipitin test, has demonstrated antibodies in almost 100 percent of patients.

Patients with this disease may also have pulmonary tuberculosis, and suitable studies should be undertaken to exclude the possibility of a double infection.

Treatment

Oral ketoconazole 200 to 400 mg daily for anything up to a year has produced total remission or sharp improvement in 96 percent of 75 cases in one study. Various forms of sulfa drug have been used in the past reasonably successfully, but sometimes resistance has developed. Cotrimoxazole (one tablet twice daily for many weeks) is probably a better treatment for patients who are not folate deficient. Amphotericin B has also been used systemically, but with the advent of ketoconazole therapy, this drug has diminished in popularity.

Follow-up

Some patients may relapse after cessation of therapy, probably because deep infection in the spleen or suprarenal does not improve as rapidly as do lesions on the skin or mucous membrane. Further experience is needed to determine wheher low doses of ketoconazole should be continued as long-term prophylactic therapy.

Selected Readings

Cuco, LC, Wroclawski, EL, Sampaio, SAP: Treatment of paracoccidioidomycosis, candidiasis, chromomycosis, lobomycosis, and mycetoma with ketoconazole. *Int J Dermatol* 1980; 19:405.

Fraga, S, Miranda, JL, Marques, A: Clinical pathological study of oral lesions in South American blastomycosis. *Cutis* 1974; 14:555.

Furtado, R: Infection versus disease in South American blastomycosis. *Int J Dermatol* 1975; 14:117.

Furtado, TA, Wilson, JW, Plunkett, OA: South American blastomycosis or paracoccidioidomycosis: The mycosis of Jutz, Splendore, and Almeida. *AMA Arch Dermatol Syphilol* 1954; 70:166.

Paracoccidioidomycosis. Proceedings of the first Pan American symposium, Washington, DC, Pan American Health Organization, 1972.

CHAPTER 19

Lobo's Disease

This deep fungal disease, which seems to have affinities with North American blastomycosis and with paracoccidioidomycosis, was first recorded by Lobo in a patient from the Amazon valley. In the past 50 years, some 100 cases have been reported from Brazil and Central America. Although this would imply that the infection is exceedingly rare, it has been suggested that a greater awareness of the disease would lead to many more cases being detected.

Etiology

The organism has never been satisfactorily cultured in vitro, while yeastlike cells seem to grow profusely in patients with the disease. It has been named *Loboa loboi,* and a suspension of the affected tissue injected into a hamster's footpad showed a reduplication of the cells some eight months later. As the lesions are mostly found on the exposed parts and are most often associated with a history of trauma, it is believed that, like *Blastomyces dermatitidis* and *Paracoccidiodes braziliensis,* the fungus probably lives in soil or vegetation.

There is an extraordinary report by Migaki et al that an organism visually indistinguishable from that found in Lobo's disease can produce severe granulomatous disease in the Atlantic bottle-nosed dolphin. Whether the organisms are identical will not be known until satisfactory culture methods have been devised.

Clinical Features

The disease shows grouped or isolated nodules that are usually painless, hard, and smooth, like keloids (Figure 19-1) (the disease has been known as keloidal blastomycosis), most commonly seen on the limbs and less frequently on the face. They vary in color from ivory to café-au-lait, and hyperpigmented lesions are extremely unusual. As time goes on, the nodules extend slowly and may become edematous, ulcerated, or even verrucous (Figure 19-2). Secondary lesions, usually appearing in areas easily reached by the fingers, indicate that the disease may be spread by autoinoculation.

Differential Diagnosis

In fully established cases, the lack of signs or symptoms in the mouth, lungs, or abdominal viscera completely rules out the diagnoses of North American blastomycosis or paracoccidioidomycosis. The rarity of ulceration and absence of lymphatic spread preclude the diagnosis of sporotrichosis. Probably the most easily confused of the deep fungal infections is chromomycosis, which sometimes can be differentiated only by differences in the biopsies.

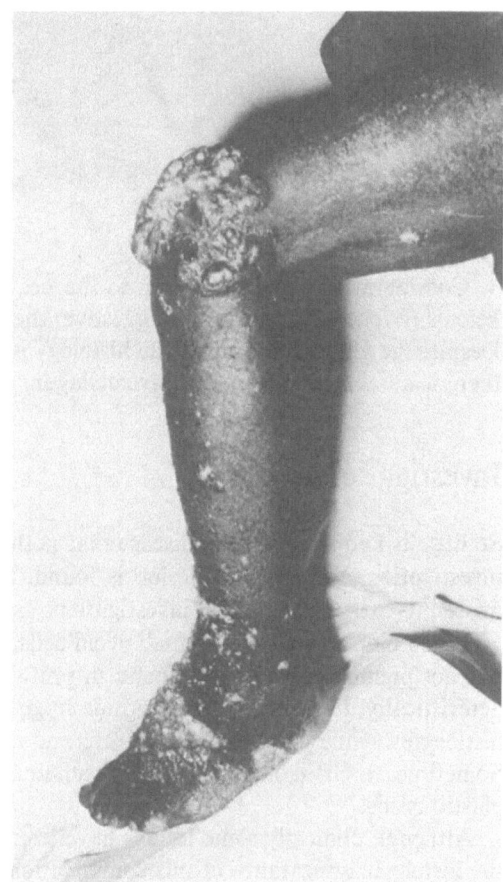

FIGURE 19-1 Granulomatous lesions resembling keloids. (Courtesy Mauricio Goihman-Yahr, M.D., Caracas, Venezuela.)

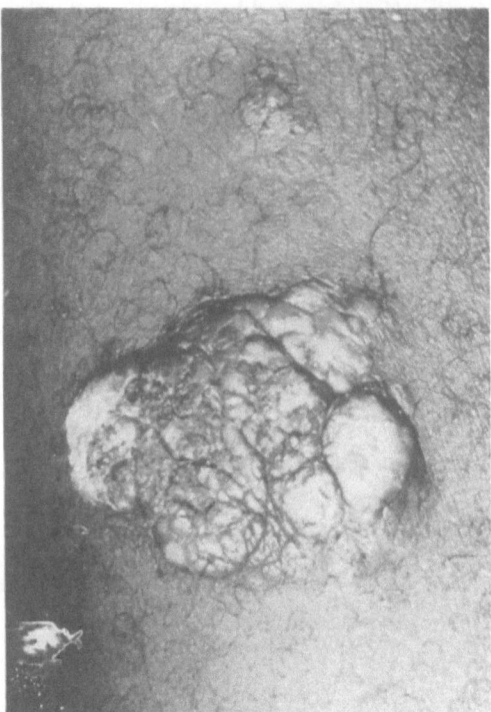

FIGURE 19-2 Elevated nodule becoming verrucous. (Courtesy J. Sidney Rice, M.D. Collection of the College of Physicians of Philadelphia.)

Consideration should be given to the possibility of hypertrophic scars and keloids. Even if the history is suggestive, the biopsy will not be confirmatory. Despite the clinical similarity, the histology is quite different; in Lobo's disease there is an absence of proliferative collagen.

Investigations

So little is known about the disease that nothing can be said about mycologic investigation. When a new lesion is found, the opportunity should never be missed to carry out as many investigations as possible.

When biopsies are taken, small ovoid cells, 7 to 10 μ in diameter, with thick but not pigmented walls, are found in profusion in granulation tissue. Characteristically, the fungi are seen inside huge foreign-body giant cells or large histiocytes, while lymphocytes are rare and collagen proliferation is not seen. Sometimes, a chain of fungal cells is seen linked to one another like a chain of plastic beads.

Although clinically some lesions have been seen to ulcerate and discharge, the histologic appearance of this complication has not been reported.

Treatment

The sparsity of cases has ensured that there are only sporadic accounts of satisfactory therapy. Clofazimine 100 mg daily and ketoconazole 400 mg daily have each shown some therapeutic success, if given for many months. Until more is known about the organism, the slowly growing, well-defined tumors are perhaps best treated by local excision.

Selected Readings

Azulay, RD, Carheiro, JA, Da Graca, M, et al: Keloid blastomycosis (Lobo's disease) with lymphatic involvement: A case report. *Int J Dermatol* 1976; 15:40.

Baruzzi, RG, Castro, RM, D'Andretta, C, et al: Occurrence of Lobo's blastomycosis among "Caiabi," Brazilian indians. *Int J Dermatol* 1973; 12:95.

Migaki, G., Valerio, MG, Irvine, B, et al: Lobo's disease in an American bottle nosed dolphin. *J Am Vet Med Assoc* 1971; 159:578.

Silva, D: Eight new cases of Lobo's keloidal mycosis. *Int J Dermatol* 1973; 12:99.

Tapia, A, Torres-Calcindo, A, Arosemena, R: Keloidal blastomycosis (Lobo's disease in Panama). *Int J Dermatol* 1978; 17:574.

PART FOUR

Parasitic Diseases

CHAPTER 20

Leishmaniasis

In different parts of the world, widely differing diseases are caused by protozoan parasites known as *Leishmania*. These parasites have two forms: they exist in human and other animals in an aflagellate state (amastigote or Leishman-Donovan bodies), while the flagellate stage (promastigote) is found in the insect vector and in culture media. The amastigote is oval or spherical and measures 2 to 6 μ in length and 1 to 2 μ in width. It is an obligate intracellular parasite. The promastigote is 15 to 25 μ long and 2 to 5 μ wide, with a flagellum that can be up to 30 μ long.

The various forms of leishmaniasis are transmitted to humans by the *Phlebotomus* sandfly and produce two different forms of clinical manifestation, the cutaneous and the visceral. It has been suspected for many years that the different types of diseases might be caused by various *Leishmania* species, but only recently have subtle differences of shape and size of the protozoa and new techniques of biochemical taxonomy given parasitologists the opportunity to produce complicated (and somewhat controversial) subdivisions of the genus.

The earliest recognized form of leishmaniasis (the Oriental sore) has been saddled with several names (Bagdad boil, Biskra button) that remind us of the areas commonly affected. The disease spreads outward from the Middle East to northeast India as far as Delhi, and along the coasts of the Mediterranean to Algeria and beyond. This type of disease is usually self-healing.

Patients whose immunologic defenses are less than complete sometimes produce a condition mimicking lupus vulgaris usually known as lupoid leishmaniasis or leishmania recidivans; others are totally unable to defend themselves against the protozoans and develop a widespread and deforming disease known as anergic leishmaniasis. In South America, some patients get an Oriental sore that later spreads to the mucocutaneous areas, producing a deforming mutilation known as mucocutaneous leishmaniasis. In India, Bangladesh, some parts of China, and Africa, patients with kala-azar (the visceral form of leish-maniasis) may later produce post-kala-azar dermal leishmaniasis.

As all these variants have different clinical presentations, are found in different parts of the world, and (probably) are caused by slightly different species of leishmania, they will each be discussed separately in the following pages.

Oriental Sore

Etiology

Leishmania tropica and its nearest relations can be found as parasites in the desert rat, dogs, and cats. The disease that they cause is limited to arid zones in which a sandfly, feeding on an infected gerbil or other reservoir host, acquires the leishmania. These will change into leishmanids (promastigotes), which, multiplying profusely in the digestive tract, are inoculated into the skin. There they are phagocytosed into histiocytes and change into leishmania (amastigotes), which multiply by binary fission. The histiocytes eventually rupture, and leishmania enter other histiocytes, leading to a pathology that, producing an Oriental sore, thus ensures that humans too can be reservoir hosts for the disease.

Leishmania major affects the gerbil and other wild desert animals and is said to be the cause of most leishmaniasis found in desert or rural areas. It is believed that *Leishmania tropica* is a natural infection of dogs and humans and is therefore more likely to cause the urban form of Oriental sore. It will of course surprise no one if patients with rural leishmaniasis are found in an urban background or vice versa.

Clinical Features

The lesion is usually solitary, appearing at the site of a sandfly bite as an itching papule somewhat erythematous and indurated, which slowly becomes crusted with thick, dark, adherent scale through which oozes a sticky serosanguinous discharge. Easily differentiable from a pyococcal infection, the nodule is painless and enlarges slowly, usually taking three to four months to attain its maximum size, which can be up to 5 cm in diameter. Most patients are loath to remove the crusted scab, as folklore persuades them that the underlying ulcer may become secondarily infected—an unwanted and painful complication. As the months go by, the ulcer begins to heal, the crusts become separated from the skin, and cicatrization starts at the center of the lesion. This will slowly spread leaving a somewhat depressed and well-defined hypopigmented scar. The whole process of infection, reaction, and spontaneous healing will take about a year; indeed in Iran it is known as *salak,* the one-year disease (Figures 20-1, 20-2).

As most lesions occur on the face, the scar can be a personal tragedy. Hypopigmented, irregular, and several centimeters in diameter, it may be so deep that men may develop cicatricial alopecia of the beard, while occasionally sores on the nostril, ear, or eyelid will cause major facial deformity (Figures 20-3, 20-4).

Natural History

Although the Oriental sore is usually solitary, sometimes a number of lesions appear at the same time. It is not known whether these are the results of numerous bites or whether there has been some endogenous spread. Such multiple lesions differ from the single sore in that they frequently show neither crusting nor ulceration.

Some authorities claim that rural leishmaniasis takes longer to run its course than does the urban variety, but this is of little practical importance, as the resultant scars are equally unwelcome. While most of the lesions sponta-

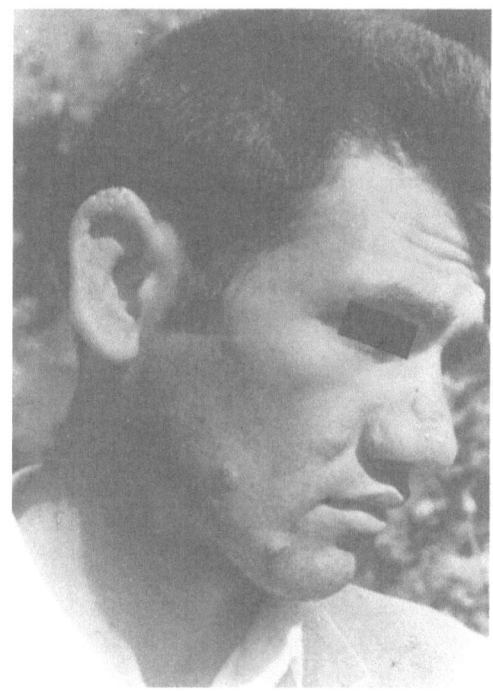

FIGURE 20-1 Several lesions of acute dermal leishmaniasis, not yet mature enough to break down and ulcerate.

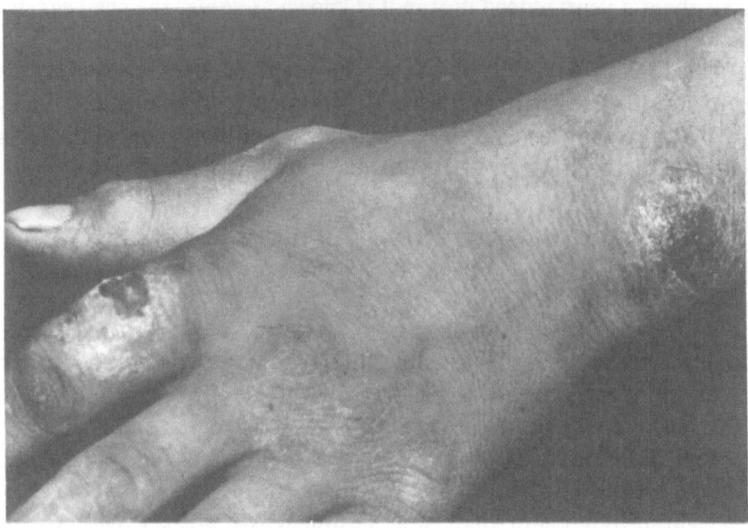

FIGURE 20-2   Ulcerating leishmaniasis on wrist and finger. (Courtesy Werner Dutz, M.D. and Efriede Kohout-Dutz, M.D., Richmond, Virginia.)

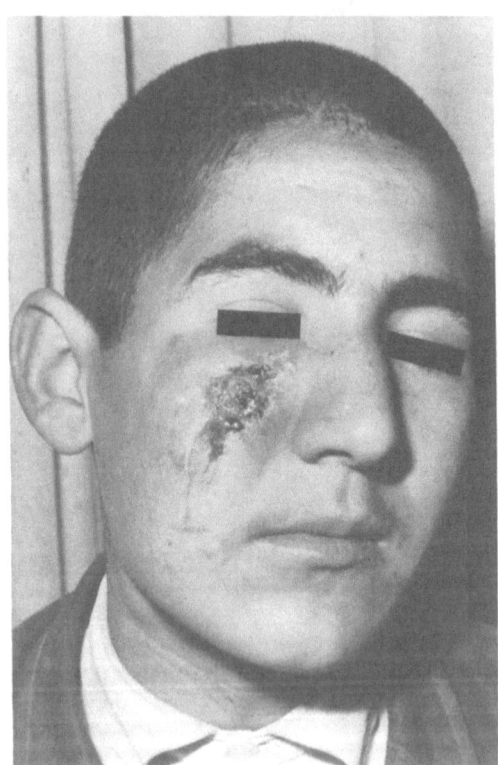

FIGURE   20-3   Leishmaniasis on the face can be associated with edema and, except for the long-standing history, might be confused with anthrax.

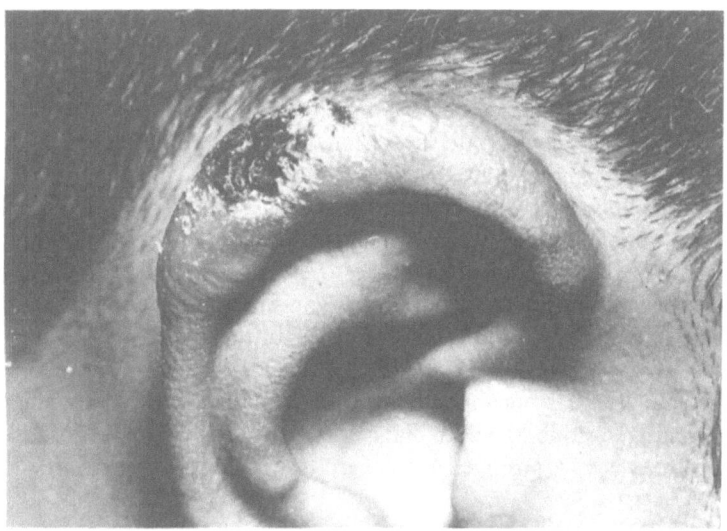

FIGURE 20-4   Oriental sore on the ear.

neously resolve, about 10 percent change their appearance and enter a different phase, described in the next section (lupoid leishmaniasis).

Differential Diagnosis

As the Oriental sore is a relatively painless, slowly developing condition that only gradually crusts and rarely ulcerates in much less than three months, it should not be difficult to differentiate it from acute bacterial diseases (boils, pyoderma, erysipelas, anthrax), which are much more rapid and usually painful.

The painless, indolent ulcer occurring in an adult who has recently visited an endemic area may be mistaken for a basal or squamous cell carcinoma, but natives of such areas usually acquire leishmaniasis in their early years, when skin malignancy is unusual.

Investigations

Intracellular parasites will be found in considerable numbers in tissue fluid either obtained by the skin-slit technique or by impression of the cut edge of a skin biopsy onto a clean glass slide. If parasites are present, material obtained by the Dutz technique (Appendix one) may be cultured at 26°C on a blood-agar medium known as NNN. Parasitologists will recognize the presence of promastigotes and the intracellular rodlike nucleus (the kinetoplast), which is described as setting a tangent to the nucleus. With the Giemsa stain, both the nucleus and kinetoplast appear bright red.

By the time a nodule has become large enough for the diagnosis to be suspected, biopsy will demonstrate the leishmania to be present in great numbers. Masses of large histiocytes are packed with organisms, which can also be seen living extracellularly. Lymphocytes and plasma cells are associated with the granuloma that underlies a somewhat proliferative epidermis. As immunity develops, the tuberculoid histology takes over, the histiocytes diminish in size and number, and in the final stages the organism cannot be found.

The leishmanin or Montenegro test is an intraepidermal test for delayed hypersensitivity. It may be of use in epidemiologic studies, but as an aid to clinical diagnosis it is not much help, being negative in the early stages and only becoming positive when the diagnosis is clinically obvious. Most adults in endemic areas have a positive Montenegro test due to an earlier infection.

Treatment

If the disease is treated early it may be possile to cause regression of infection before it has reached a stage where scarring is inevitable. Therapy is not as successful as might be hoped. Systemically pentavalent antimonials are most widely used—500 mg of sodium stibogluconate may be given, intramuscularly or intravenously, for 10 to 14 days. Attempts to treat small lesions by local intradermal injection are not to be encouraged as the residual scar is in no way different from that which follows an untreated infection. There have been scattered claims of satisfactory results from the use of amphotericin B or rifampicin, while anecdotal reports of drugs too numerous to mention have usually not been supported by further studies.

There is, however, an interesting new technique at present being investigated in which the antileishmaniasis drugs are coated with lyposomes and administered intravenously. Phagocytic cells in the skin rapidly remove lyposomes from the bloodstream, and the drug is thereby delivered directly into the histiocytes that contain the infecting organism. It is not yet known whether these experiments can lead to a clinically useful therapy.

Small lesions can be surgically excised or destroyed by electrosurgery or cryosurgery. These techniques are particularly useful as a method of limiting extension of infection of the nostril or ear.

Parents living in endemic areas believe patients are never infected twice and frequently seek for their child, particularly if it is a girl, to be vaccinated in a covered area, preferring a scar on the buttock or thigh to one on the face. It is now believed that *L. major* (cause of the rural disease) will protect against *L. tropica,* but the opposite is not necessarily true.

While there is no harm in such vaccination in the Old World, it should not be recommended in South America, as inoculation with *L. braziliensis* may be followed by mucocutaneous leishmaniasis.

Lupoid Leishmaniasis

More than 90 percent of all patients who have Oriental sore overcome the infection totally at the expense of developing an unsightly scar. Sometimes, however, as the crust falls away from the healing ulcer the patient finds active nodules still present in the skin. Less frequently, the sore heals completely and nodules appear in the scar some time later. This is the start of the condition that has varyingly been called chronic leishmaniasis, lupoid leishmaniasis, or leishmaniasis cutis recidivans.

Clinical Features

Scattered throughout the scar are many yellowish-brown translucent nodules of the apple-jelly type over which the skin is thinned. Sometimes these nodules develop on an erythematous or hyperpigmented background and gradually spread peripherally, causing the original scar to extend and producing a picture that is indistinguishable from lupus vulgaris. In a surprising number of cases in Iran the patient gives a history of seasonal variation in the lesions and expects them to get worse in summer. It is not unusual to find that nodules have ulcerated after exposure to sunshine (Figures 20-5 to 20-7).

Natural History

The Oriental sore takes about a year to run its course. Only in the last stages is it recognized that some patients are not going to heal normally. There is little or no tendency for this form of leishmaniasis to regress. In one series of nearly 70 cases all the patients had had the disease for at least eight years, since acute cutaneous disease had at that time been eradicated, when the sandflies were fortuitously exterminated during an antimalarial compaign.

Differential Diagnosis

It is extremely difficult to differentiate this from lupus vulgaris if the patient does not relate that the condition started with an Oriental sore. In endemic areas, such a history is usually available, as the patients are well aware of the clinical appearance of primary cutaneous leishmaniasis. If, in sporadic cases seen elsewhere, this information is not available, the diagnosis may indeed be difficult to establish. It may even be necessary to treat the patient with anti-tuberculosis therapy for a few months: if there is not a dramatic improvement, leishmaniasis may be suspected.

Except for other causes of tuberculoid granulomata, no other disease need be considered in the differential diagnosis.

Investigations

Smears taken from an acute Oriental sore abound with leishmania, and culture produces large numbers of the leptomonad form. This does not apply to lupoid leishmaniasis, where it is suspected that the body's attempt to eradicate infection by production of a cell-mediated immunity is less than totally successful, and (comparable to tuberculoid leprosy or lupus vulgaris) a spreading tuberculoid granuloma shows that immunity, although high, is not complete. Attempts to culture organisms from such granulomata are met with scanty success. In most patients it is impossible to obtain a positive culture.

Similarly unhelpful are attempts to confirm the diagnosis histologically. The tuberculoid granuloma is indistinguishable from those found in tuberculosis or the tuberculoid form of leprosy. Caseation has never been reported in lupoid leishmaniasis and if seen will rule out the diagnosis. An associated hypertrophy of the epidermis amounting almost to pseudoepitheliomatous hyperplasia can produce a histologic appearance similar to that found in chromomycosis, but without the diagnostic thick-walled intracellular spores.

In most cases, the Montenegro test is positive. This is useful in children, but not much help diagnostically in areas where almost all adults have a positive reaction. In cases where the disease afflicts a person who has only fleetingly visited an endemic area, a positive Montenegro test and a negative tuberculin test may combine to suggest the diagnosis.

Treatment

Physicians with experience in the Middle East will know that the treatment of chronic leishmaniasis is depressingly unsuccessful. Spontaneous cure cannot be expected, and prolonged courses of the usual pentavalent antimonials must be tried. Intravenous pentostam is the treatment of choice, supplemented if possible with grenz rays every two to three weeks.

In smaller lesions, the individual apple-jelly nodules may be treated with liquid phenol or 20 percent trichloracetic acid. The granulomas may be destroyed in this way, and the resultant cicatrization will not be worse than that produced by the disease. Cryotherapy can also be used.

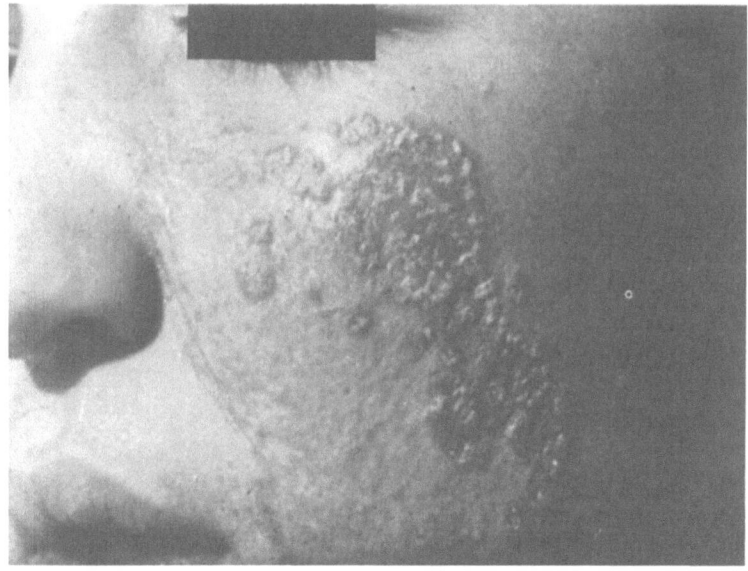

FIGURE 20-5   Lupoid leishmaniasis (resembling lupus vulgaris).

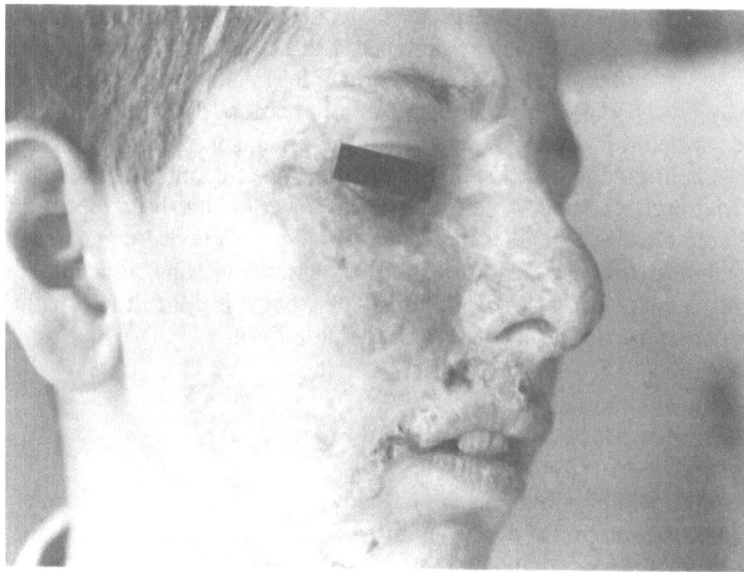

FIGURE 20-6   Lupoid leishmaniasis extending widely over the face.

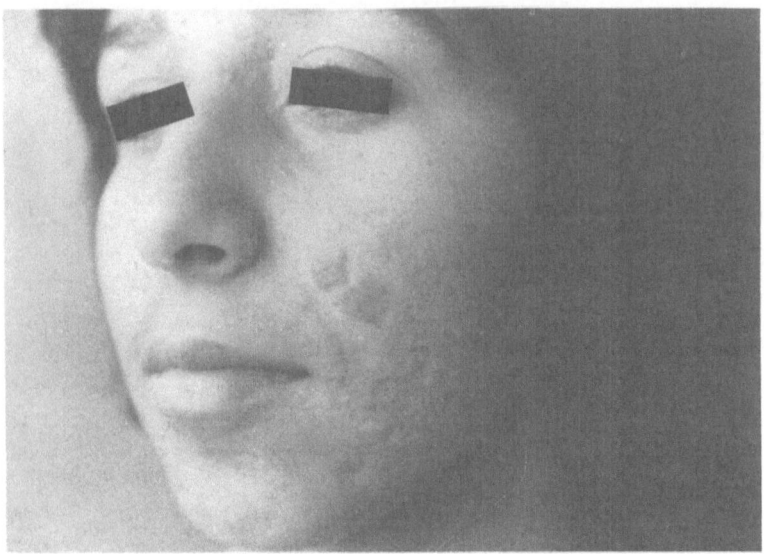

FIGURE 20-7   Acute leishmaniasis left a scar on the left cheek. One year later new apply-jelly nodules appeared and are enlarging.

Anergic Leishmaniasis

The Oriental sore is found mainly in the Middle East and around the borders of the Mediterranean. Lupoid leishmaniasis, although less frequent, appears in much the same sites. There is another form of leishmaniasis in which the entire skin may be covered with nodules, apparently because patients are completely unable to mount a defensive reaction to the organism. Diffuse anergic leishmaniasis is limited to central Africa (Ethiopia, the Sudan, Tanzania) and the equatorial parts of South America. It seems never to have been reported from the Middle East, but whether these geographic preferences are manifestations of immunologic differences in the protozoa or in the varying susceptibilities of the hosts is unknown. It is probably the latter, but it is difficult to explain why such a defect has not been noted in the Middle East.

Clinical Features

Lesions of lupoid leishmaniasis are in many ways comparable to those of tuberculoid leprosy, except of course leprosy granulomata invade the nerves as well as the dermis. In a similar way, patients who are anergic to leishmaniasis develop a widespread abnormality that is comparable in almost every way to lepromatous leprosy; the condition has sometimes been called leproid leishmaniasis.

When the condition is fully established, there is a symmetrical eruption of soft bulky nodules on the face and ears with others all over the extremities; the trunk is less frequently involved. Many lesions resemble soft, shiny keloids, but others are somewhat scaly or even have a verrucosus surface (Figures 20-5 to 20-7). The outer parts of the eyebrows are missing (madarosis), and patients may complain of dryness of the nose or epistaxis, but although the mucosa is often erythematous, intranasal nodules are rarely found. In contrast to lepromatous leprosy, the skin between the lesions not only looks normal, but contains no leishmania.

Natural History

In most cases the disease starts with a small, painless nodule on an exposed part. This is probably the site of inoculation by a sandfly, but the progress usual in an Oriental sore does not take place. The nodule enlarges but neither ulcerates nor crusts, and after a few months satellite lesions develop around the primary one. Over the years a variety of nodules appears all over the body. In about 20 percent of cases the primary lesion heals, leaving the patient's skin completely normal for a few months, after which extensive numbers of papules erupt and enlarge in the classical sites. This temporary healing suggests that these patients are not primarily anergic, but that their low degree of immunologic defense collapses under the weight of protozoal multiplication and they become secondarily anergic.

The onset of the disease is not infrequently associated with a period of general malaise, but after a few years general symptoms are not seen unless the patient has entered a phase in which the existing lesions become red and swollen in a manner that is exactly comparable to the clinical appearance of leprosy patients in reaction. Records of such happenings are unclear as to whether these events are associated with subsequent clinical improvement, analogous to a reversal reaction.

Differential Diagnosis

Many of these patients have been found living in the world's leprosaria often diagnosed as having abacterial lepromatous leprosy. Widespread lymphoma may often cause diagnostic confusion while sarcoidosis and extensive keloids may also be suspected. The histology should always clarify matters.

Investigations

These patients are full of leishmania. Abundant parasites can be found in skin smears, while culture on the NNN medium is profusely successful. If a biopsy is taken, the epidermis is normal or mildly thickened, and there is a dense dermal infiltrate consisting of numerous vacuolated histiocytes looking like the foam cells of lepromatous leprosy, but containing masses of parasites that are easily demonstrated by the Giemsa stain. Lymphocytes and plasma cells are mixed with the infiltrate, but the granuloma never involves cutaneous nerves.

In anergic patients the Montenegro test is invariably negative. It has been said that any case diagnosed as lepromatous leprosy in Ethiopia that does not show acid-fast bacilli should be examined for leishmania; this rule applies throughout the world.

Treatment

These unfortunate individuals have inherited the grim prognosis that used to be given for lepromatous leprosy before the use of sulfones. Of the usual antimonials, diamidinophenoxypentane (pentamidine) is probably the drug of choice, but it must be used very carefully because in cases of gross disease a form of Herxheimer's reaction has been seen.

Rifampicin alone or supplemented with isoniazid or sodium stibogluconate can be tried; amphotericin B and ketoconazole have also been used. The fact remains that most of these patients do not respond to any known form of therapy.

Mucocutaneous Leishmaniasis

Leishmania braziliensis is one of the 13 known forms of leishmania recognized in South America alone. It can be found in such wild animals as the marmoset and racoon, particularly those inhabiting the forest areas of the Andes. It produces in humans a disfiguring disease known as mucocutaneous leishmaniasis, found mainly in South America. Brazil, Venezuela, and Peru have the most cases.

Variants of *Leishmania braziliensis* have been named after the countries in which they were first detected.

Clinical Features

Although any mucocutaneous site may be involved, including the anus or vulva, the classical form affects the nasal passages, where redness, induration, and infiltration lead to a destructive lesion referred to as a camel's nose or

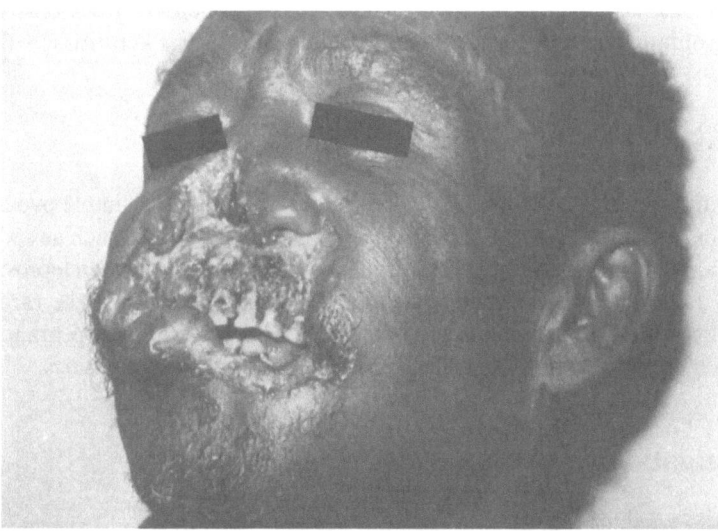

FIGURE 20-8   Late necrotizing granuloma of mucocutaneous leishmaniasis called espundia. (Courtesy J. Sidney Rice, M.D. Collection of the College of Physicians of Philadelphia.)

parrot's beak. Swelling followed by destruction starts in the nasal septum and extends out to the upper lip and back to the nasal-pharyngeal passage. Later the tongue, buccal mucosa, and floor of the mouth can be destroyed as the condition extends to other parts of the face (Figure 20-8). In the later stages, infection may metastasize to other parts of the body.

Sepsis frequently complicates matters; the patient can become malnourished because of difficulties in eating, and respiratory failure can follow obstruction of the bronchotracheal passage and secondary infection of the lung.

Natural History

The classical picture of destructive involvement of the nose and face is not the beginning of the story since this condition starts as a tropical sore that may be sited on any part of the skin and runs much the same course as similar lesions in other parts of the world. The condition caused by *L. braziliensis* varies from other forms of leishmaniasis in that anything from a few days to 25 years after the start of the original infection secondary lesions develop in one or more mucocutaneous junctions. Most often this extension starts with what the patient thinks is a chronic cold or epistaxis, later, the nasal cartilage becomes involved, the nose collapses, and the classic midfacial destruction develops.

Further extension can even reach the eye, causing granulomatous destruction of the conjunctiva with corneal ulceration and intersititial keratitis.

Differential Diagnosis

Many diseases give a similar clinical picture, starting with a simple pyoderma, rhinophyma, rhinoscleroma, and various deep fungal diseases such as sporotrichosis and paracoccidiodomycosis. Lupus vulgaris, yaws, and even leprosy produce a somewhat similar (but less extensive) destruction, while the rare condition known as lethal midline granuloma may have a similar appearance.

The diagnosis cannot be confirmed without suitable investigations.

Investigations

This may be looked on as a disease midway between lupoid and anergic leishmaniasis. Although leishmania are not difficult to detect they are neither as rare as they are in lupoid disease nor as profuse as in anergic infection. The simplest method is to use a skin smear similar to that used to demonstrate *Mycobacterium leprae* (see Appendix one) and stain the tissue fluid with Giemsa, Wright's, or Leishman's stains. As with leprosy smears it is important to ensure that the smear is not heavily contaminated with blood, in which case the relatively rare amastigotes may be missed. As in other forms of leishmaniasis, culture can be achieved in the Nicolle-Novy-MacNeal (NNN) agar. The Montegro test is not much use as not all patients are positive, and many normal people in the region react because of previous exposure.

Biopsy of the erosion will show a necrotizing tuberculoid granuloma that is only differentiable from lupus vulgaris, leprosy, etc. by virtue of the presence of the protozoa. As these are relatively scanty it is often necessary to examine several sections before the diagnosis can be confirmed.

Various serologic tests are known, but are of more value as research tools than as aids to diagnosis.

Treatment

The condition almost never heals by itself without massive destruction. The important treatments include the pentavalent antimonial compounds, but a competent immune system is necessary for any of the drugs to work satisfactorily. The most useful is *N*-methylglucamine antimoniae, which is given 100 mg per day for 20 days, but it has a fairly high failure rate. An alternative sodium stibogluconate may be needed. It is given intramuscularly daily for two to three weeks.

Alternatively, amphotericin B can be given intravenously at an initial dose of 0.5 mg/kg every three to four hours, gradually raised to 10 mg/kg until a maximum of 2,5000 to 3,000 mg has been given.

Most recently, ketoconazole 400 mg orally for at least three months has proved itself a well-tolerated and easily administered modality.

Cryosurgery is useful and rational, as the organisms are known to be sensitive to temperature changes.

There is no known way to immunize people living in endemic areas. The best hope for prophylaxis is for extensive public health campaigns to eradicate the sandfly.

Post-Kala-Azar Dermal Leishmaniasis

Kala-azar is the name usually given to a visceral infection caused by *Leishmania donovani*. Not uncommon in northeastern Brazil but found more frequently in central Africa, the borders of the Mediterranean, and parts of Russia, India, Bangladesh, and China, the established disease shows enormous hepatosplenomegaly with recurrent fever and a progressive wasting, which, in fair-skinned patients, is associated with darkening of the skin (kala-azar is Hindi for "the black fever").

Clinical Features

Some 3 to 30 months after they have had kala-azar some of these patients develop dermatologic lesions of almost infinite variety. Hypopigmented macules, nodules, pseudoxanthomata, verrucose lesions, and a sort of proliferative condylomata have all been reported. Many of these patients are mistakenly treated for leprosy despite the absence of acid-fast bacilli or of any neurologic signs.

A butterfly erythema, aggravated by sunlight, may be the earliest sign, slowly followed by the development of hypopigmented macules covering the whole body. Later, nodules appear, mainly on the face and ears, that with time become more disseminated, taking on a warty or even verrucose appearance (Figures 20-9a,b to 20-11).

Natural History

Kala-azar is becoming a rare disease in most parts of the world, because attempts to eradicate the sandfly have been successful in many places. In India, post-kala-azar dermal leishmaniasis is probably now more common than kala-azar itself, as, once established, the lesions tend to persist or extend for many years.

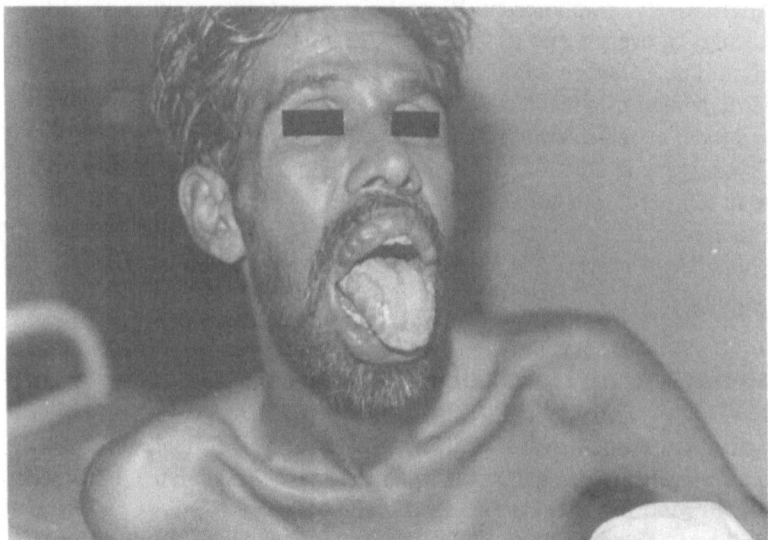

a

b

FIGURE 20-9a,b   A case of pulmonary thuberculosis referred for hoarseness of voice
with swelling of lip and tongue for six months. The smear of Leishman-Donovan bodies was positive from lip, tongue, and larynx.

FIGURE 20-10 Nodules on nose being treated as rosacea. The smear was positive for Leishman-Donovan bodies.

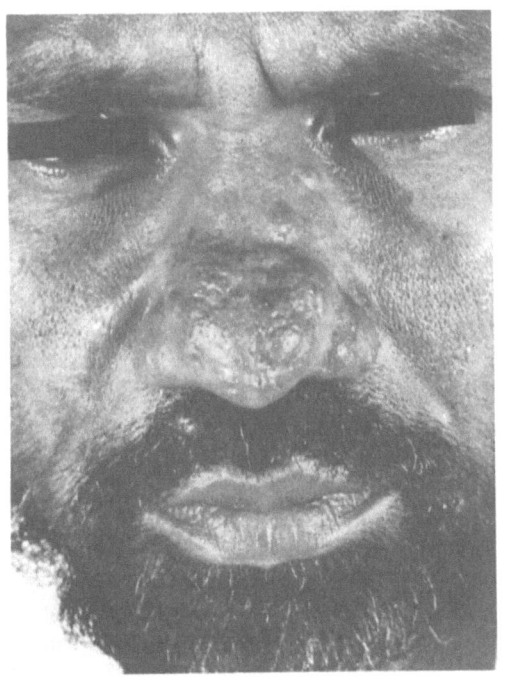

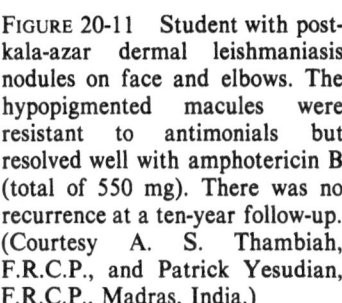

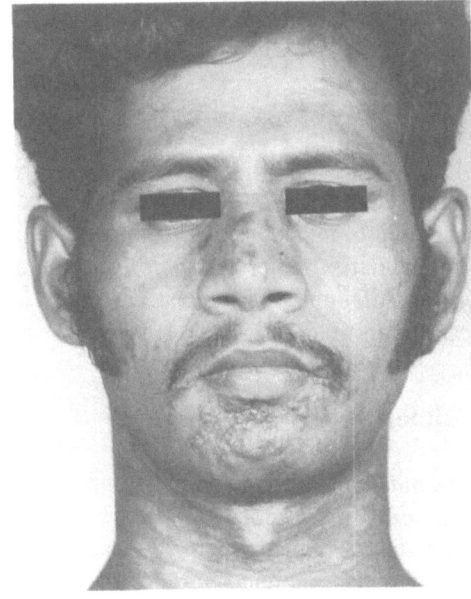

FIGURE 20-11 Student with post-kala-azar dermal leishmaniasis nodules on face and elbows. The hypopigmented macules were resistant to antimonials but resolved well with amphotericin B (total of 550 mg). There was no recurrence at a ten-year follow-up. (Courtesy A. S. Thambiah, F.R.C.P., and Patrick Yesudian, F.R.C.P., Madras, India.)

This symptom complex is probably a manifestation of immunologic insufficiency and does not occur in all cases of visceral disease, since most patients will have some resistance to infection.

Differential Diagnosis

Any form of leprosy may be mimicked by this condition. A previous history of kala-azar will be helpful, but it is not obtained in many cases. Moreover, there is of course no reason why, in infected areas, a patient with leprosy cannot also have a prevous history of kala-azar.

This wide variety of lesions can easily confuse the clinician, but the presence of firm granulomatous lesions around the mouth and nose and a scattering of hypopigmented macules elsewhere should be of assistance.

Investigations

In the macular form the causative organisms are frequently not detectable, but they are present in good numbers in the nodular forms of disease, in which case positive skin smears stained by Giemsa stain will be enough to confirm the histology, but if a biopsy is taken it will usually show a histology similar to that seen in anergic disease with a heavy infiltrate of histiocytes containing numerous parasites.

As usual, the Montenegro test is of little value, as it may or may not be positive.

Treatment

As may be expected, if the disease is limited to the macular form it will respond fairly well to injections of stibophen (2 ml intramuscularly on alternate days). The nodular varieties are more resistant to antimonials, but may respond to hydroxystilbamidine isothionate. Amphotericin B therapy has been used successfully in Madras.

Chiclero's Ulcer

Leishmania mexicana is usually found on the east coast of Mexico and Central America. The lesion it causes is similar to an ordinary Oriental sore, but usually lasts less than six months. If, as is not unusual, the lesion affects the ear, the infection commonly invades the cartilage and produces a severe erosive deformity that shows little tendency to spontaneous resolution.

By far, the best treatment is destruction of the lesion with electrosurgery or cryosurgery, thus terminating the usual inexorable spread.

Pian Bois

Leishmania braziliensis guyanensis infection produces numerous lesions on the body that, unlike most Oriental sores, show a sporotrichoid tendency to spread along the lymphatics and even to infect the regional lymph nodes. The nose and mouth are not involved.

Selected Readings

Chance, ML: Leishmaniasis. *Br Med J* 1981; 283:1245.

Connor, DH, Neafie, RC: Cutaneous leishmaniasis, in Binford, CH, Connor, DH (eds): *Pathology of Tropical and Extraordinary Diseases.* Washington, DC, Armed Forces Institute of Pathology, 1976, p 258.

Convit, J, Kerdel-Vegas, F, Gordon, B: Disseminated anergic leishmaniasis. *Br J Dermatol* 1962; 74:132.

Kerdel-Vegas, F: American leishmaniasis. *Int J Dermatol* 1982; 21:291.

Kern, P: Leishmaniasis antibiotics. *Chemotherapy* 1981; 30:203.

Lainson, R: The American leishmaniasis: Some observations on their ecology and epidemiology. *R Soc Trop Med Hyg* 1983; 77:569.

The Leishmaniac: A Periodical. Jerusalem, Kuvin Centre for the Study of Infectious and Tropical Diseases.

Munro, DD, du Vivier, A, Jopling,WH: Post-kala-azar dermal leishmaniasis. *Br J Dermatol* 1972; 87:374.

Pareek, SS: Combination therapy of sodium stibogluconate and rifampin in cutaneous leishmaniasis. Int J Dermatol 1984; 23:70.

Pettit, JHS: Chronic (lupoid) leishmaniasis. *Br J Dermatol* 1962; 74:127.

Sagher, F: Some basic medical problems illustrate by experiments with cutaneous leishmaniasis. *Trans St. John's Hosp Dermatol Soc* 1972; 58:1.

Schewach-Millet, M, Fisher, BK, Semah, D: Leishmaniasis recidivans treated with sodium stibogluconate. *Cutis* 1981; 28:67.

Strick, RA, Borok, M, Basiorowski HC: Recurrent cutaneous leishmaniasis. J Am Acad Dermatol 983; 9:437.

Turk, JL: Leprosy and leishmaniasis. *Proc R Soc Med* 1970; 63:1053.

Weinrauch, L, Lirshin, R, Even-Pas, Z, et al: Efficacy of ketoconazole in cutaneous leishmaniasis. *Arch Dermatol Res* 1983; 275:353.

Urcuyo, FG, Zaias, N: Oral ketoconazole in the treatment of leishmaniasis. *Int J Dermatol* 1982; 21:414.

Yesudian, P, Thambiah, AS: Amphotericin B therapy in dermal leishmanoid. *Arch Dermatol* 1974; 109:720.

CHAPTER 21

Amebiasis

Amebiasis is an infection of the gastrointestinal tract, usually the colon, that may remain localized for many years. At any time, this protozoan infection can spread to other parts of the lower intestine, the liver, and even additional internal organs, where it is not unusual for abscesses to form. Cutaneous amebiasis is the result of extension of these abscesses to nearby skin; direct inoculation may also produce an amebic ulcer. Both sexes are infected, and there is no age limit. The duration of the disease varies from a few weeks to several years. Cutaneous amebiasis occurs worldwide—it is not necessarily limited to third-world countries, but can even be found in major American metropolitan areas. It is, however, more common in those parts of the third world where little attention is paid to sanitation.

Etiology

The condition was first recognized a century ago. It is caused by the protozoan *Entamoeba histolytica*. This parasite can exist in two forms: the cyst (10 to 20μ in diameter) and the trophozoite (12 to $50\ \mu$). Both can be found in dogs, cats, and rabbits, which are known reservoirs of the infection.

Human beings contract the disease by ingesting cysts from contaminated water or food fertilized with night soil. Trophozoites excyst in the small intestine and enter the colon, where they invade the mucosa. Individuals may have a few lesions, often asymptomatic, but other patients may be more susceptible and develop a severe infection. This is probably limited to those in whom malnutrition combines with decreased immunologic competence. The trophozoites, under certain circumstances, encyst, leave the body, and complete the cycle.

Infection may spread to the liver, where single or multiple cysts develop varying sizes, containing amorphous necrotic material. These abscesses may track to the skin, overlying the liver, or sometimes spread to the flank, where they ulcerate. Ulcers may also occur in the perineum by extension from a rectal or vaginal infection and have also been reported to arise *de novo* on the penis; in the last instance, both heterosexual and homosexual contacts are thought to play a role in transmission.

Clinical Features

The most common symptom of amebic infection is bloody diarrhea. but this is not always seen. Jaundice or an enlarged, painful liver may be the first clinical manifestation. Extraintestinal infection may produce such nonspecific symptoms as malaise and fever. It is not unknown for a cutaneous lesion to develop in a patient whose intestinal and hepatic infection have not been recognized. It may start with mild itching, but soon definite pain is felt and the skin breaks down to form an irregular ulcer with a sharply defined border. This may be masked by overgrowth of granulation tissue or even covered with a necrotic eschar. The picture can be complicated by the appearance of a nonspecific sensitizing eruption (an amebid lesion), which is an allergic type of response to the underlying *Entamoeba,* but in which no organisms can be found.

Natural History

Trophozoites lodging in the intestine will usually cause features of amebic dysentery within a few days; the distended abdomen, associated with mucoid or bloody diarrhea, may persist for months or years if it is untreated, but other patients may remain undiagnosed for years, particularly if nonspecific abdominal symptoms alternate with periods of relatively good health.

The extension of underlying infection onto the skin causes a painful ulcer, which extends rapidly with a malodorous necrotic base (Figures 21-1 to 21-3). Sometimes, the edges produce a warty proliferation, when pseudoepitheliomatous hypertrophy develops at the edge of the ulcer. It is most unlikely that these ulcers will heal spontaneously.

Differential Diagnosis

Other causes of rapidly extending cutaneous ulceration must be excluded; tuberculous and syphilitiz ulcers are usually painless. Lesions on the penis can be confused with chancroid, but the most difficult problem is differentiating

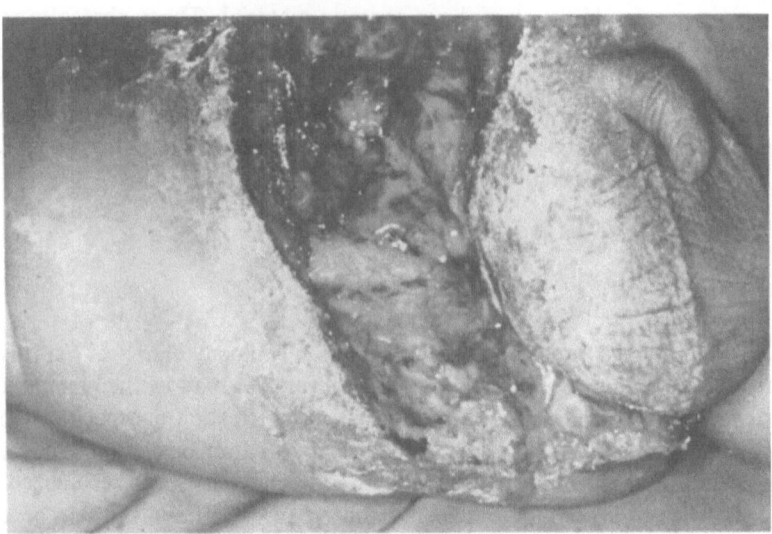

FIGURE 21-1   Painful ulceration of the groin. (Courtesy Liverpool School of Tropical Medicine, England.)

this from pyoderma gangrenosum. Condylomata acuminata, skin malignancies, and the deep mycoses are among the wide variety of warty lesions that can be confused with the hypertrophic cauliflowerlike reaction surrounding the ulcer. All of these diagnoses can be disproved by demonstration of the *Entamoeba* in the tissues.

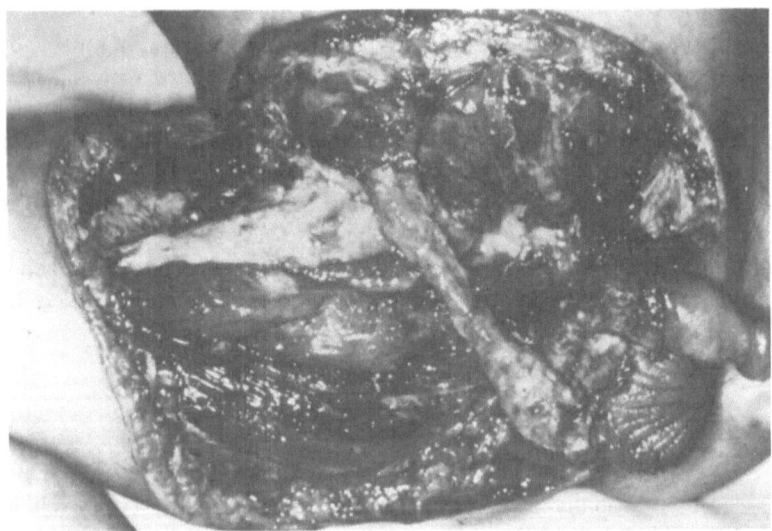

FIGURE 21-2   Closer view reveals the extensive necrosis. (Courtesy Liverpool School of Tropical Medicine, England.)

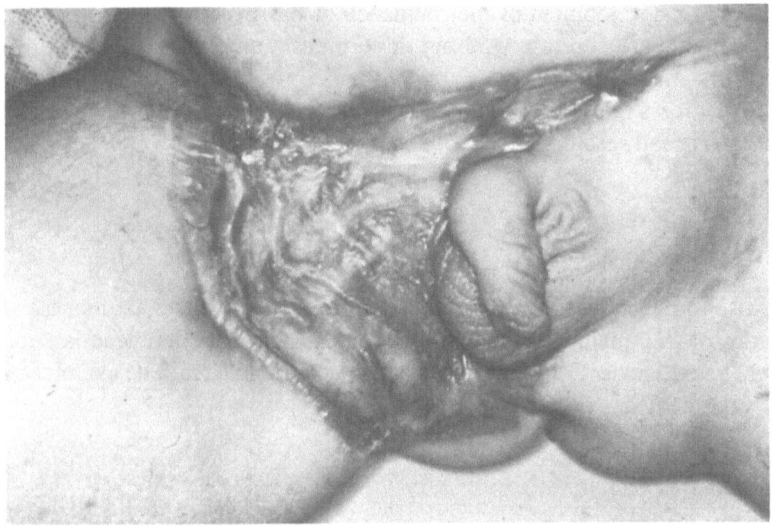

FIGURE 21-3   Marked destruction extending onto the perineal area. Note the hyper-trophic margins. (Courtesy Liverpool School of Tropical Medicine, England.)

Investigations

Although the diagnosis of cutaneous amebiasis may often be made simply by clinical inspection, it is wise to seek the trophozoites in the discharge as well as in the stools. If this is not successful, biopsy from the edge of the necrotic part of the ulcer will usually contain trophozoites that are readily stainable with hematoxylin and eosin.

If these are not seen in a skin section, the diagnosis will probably not be made histologically, as the other changes are nonspecific, with necrosis associated with lymphocytes and plasma cells somewhat complicated by benign epidermal proliferation.

A skin test with axenic-amebic antigen will produce a tuberculoid type of reaction in about 80 percent of cases. Complement-fixation tests, hemagglutination, indirect immunofluorescence, immunophoresis, and agar gel diffusion tests, available in some centers, are usually helpful.

Treatment

In the past, various methods of treatment have been reasonably successful.

Chloroquine 600 mg daily for ten weeks along with 650 mg diiodohydroxyquin three times a day for three weeks can be used. Dihydroemetine (1 mg/kg intramuscularly daily for ten days) can be used alone or in combination with chloroquine.

Since the development of metronidazole it has become the drug of choice. Most patients are cured by 750 mg three times a day (20 to 50 mg/kg) for 7 to 21 days.

Large ulcers may show so much necrosis that surgical debridement is necessary to spread resolution.

Follow-up

It is wise to check the feces for *Entameba* at one month and six months after cessation of treatment. It should also be remembered that cutaneous amebiasis is highly contagious. Other members of the household should be examined and their stools tested.

Selected Readings

Biagi, F: Amebiasis. *Antibiot Chemother* 1981; 30:20.
Krogstad, DJ, Spencer, HC, Healy, GR: Current concepts in parasitology: Amebiasis. *N Engl J Med* 1978; 298:262.
Padilla, CA, Padilla, GM: *Amebiasis in Man.* Springfield, Ill, Charles C Thomas, 1974.
Saúl, A: Amoebiasis cutis. *Int J Dermatol* 1982; 21:472.
Symposium on amebiasis. *Bull NY Acad Med,* 2nd ser 1981; 57:173.

CHAPTER 22

Toxoplasmosis

This potentially devastating disease can be found in most areas of the world. It is believed that more than one billion sufferers exist in North and South America, Australia, and Asia. It is also found in Europe to such an extent that at least 50 percent of the population of Italy is said to have toxoplasmosis, but because the infection often remains subclinical, it often is unrecognized.

Etiology

The causative organism is a coccidian parasite that may live in domestic or farm animals, although the cat is most usually blamed. *Toxoplasma gondii* is 5 μ in length and appears as a crescent with a rounded end. This organism undergoes schizogony and gametogony in intestinal epithelium and is most commonly found as an intracellular organism in the nervous, muscular, or reticuloedothelial systems.

The mechanism of transmission is uncertain, but because there is a more frequent incidence among butchers and veterinarians, it is believed that direct transmission from infected animal tissue is possible. Cats, rats, dogs, cattle, pigs, sheep, and fowl are all known to pass cysts and pseudocysts through the feces. The disease has also been acquired from eating fresh, uncooked meat.

Infected women have been known to excrete toxoplasma in their menstrual blood, lochial secretion, maternal milk, and amniotic fluid and so are a source of intrauterine toxoplasmosis with its triad of symptoms—hydrocephalus, chorioretinitis, and calcification of the brain. In older children, the central nervous system is chiefly affected by meningitis and encephalitis. In adults the viscera are most frequently affected, while airborne transmission probably explains the occasional appearance of lesions in the lung.

Clinical Features

Most patients have few or no symptoms. Unfortunately, if the skin is involved, the morphologic picture of cutaneous toxoplasmosis is generally so nonspecific that it does not help the diagnosis. There may be a diffuse morbilliform eruption either alone or associated with scattered macules and papules. Purpura, petechiae, erythema multiforme (Figure 22-1), and scaliness may all be seen, and gumma formation, nodules, and cysts occur in the later stages (Figure 22-2).

Natural History

The natural history is always difficult to determine in a disease which is either asymptomatic or produces only a vague symptomatology. In the noncongenital form, during the first few weeks of infection, a transient maculopapular eruption is seen. Later, malaise, arthralgia, headache, and fever begin. Immuno-suppressed patients are more susceptible and may develop a fulminant infection: tachycardia, febrile episodes, pneumonitis, and inflammation of the myocardium, the meninges, and the gastrointestinal tract can combine to cause their death.

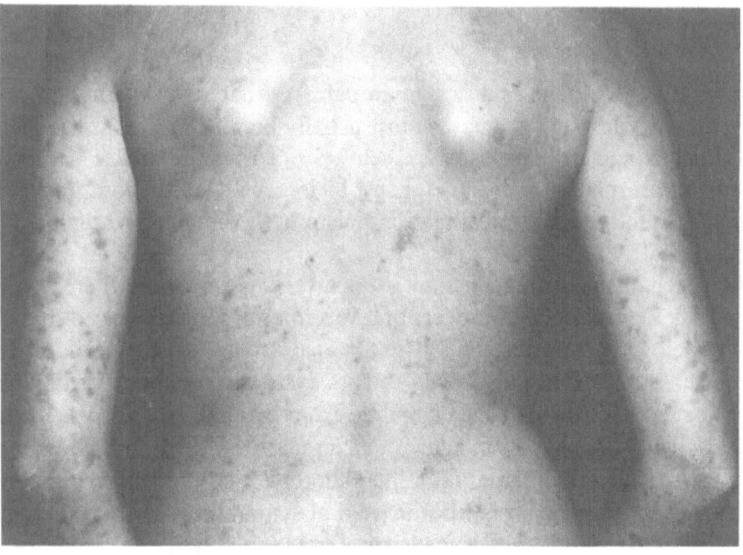

FIGURE 22-1 Erythema multiforme-like eruption in an 18-year-old Italian woman. (Courtesy Maurizio Binazzi, M.D., Perugia, Italy.)

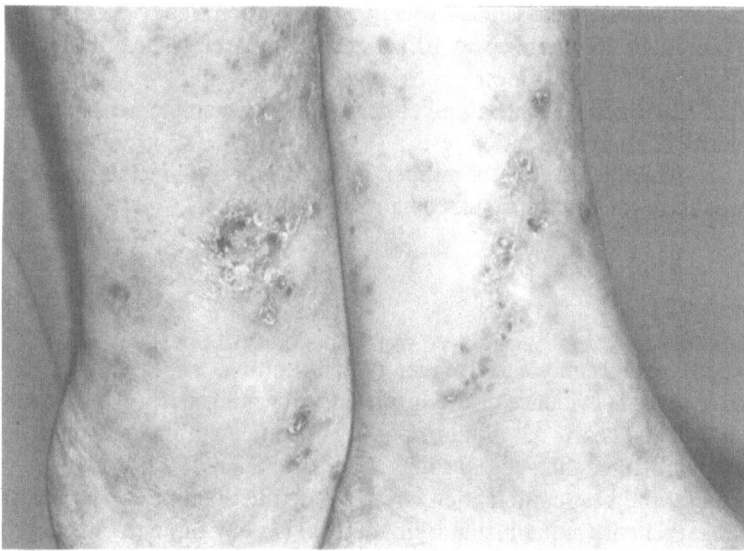

FIGURE 22-2   Nodules and crusting on the legs of a 61-year-old Italian woman. (Courtesy Maurizio Binazzi, M.D., Perugia, Italy.)

Although most cases are self-limiting, the disease can take a chronic course, in which case nodules and cysts finally appear in the skin, particularly on the scalp.

Differential Diagnosis

Fever, vague skin eruptions, and neurologic signs may be confused with tick-borne typhus or meningococcal meningitis. It must also be remembered that toxoplasmosis is one of the causes of generalized lymphadenopathy. Cutaneous lymphomas, dermatomyositis, and lichen planus all at various times can confuse the diagnostically unwary.

Investigations

Organisms are easily recognized in biopsies from infected tissue, as they stain nicely with methylene blue. Aside from these, the lesion shows nothing but a nonspecific inflammatory reaction.

The presence of toxoplasma does not indicate whether the infection is recent or long-standing. It is necessary to resort to serologic tests, of which the indirect fluorescent antibody test is most widely used. High antibody titers suggest an acute infection, although up to 10 percent of apparently healthy individuals may also show high readings.

Other tests include the Sabin-Feldman dye test, complement-fixation test, and indirect hemagglutination tests.

If it is available, 0.1 mg of antigen injected into an infected patient's skin will produce a flare with pseudopodia within 30 minutes.

Treatment

Cutaneous toxoplasmosis is frequently self-limiting, and treatment is only needed if there is evidence of eye involvement or other deep manifestations in the brain or the heart. All immunologically incompetent patients must also be treated. Unfortunately, success cannot be guaranteed.

Probably the best combination is to give pyrimethamine 25 mg four times a day together with sulfadiazine 1 gm four times a day for many weeks. Unfortunately, adverse reactions to the folate antagonist are relatively common.

Other treatments reported to be successful include tetracycline in various doses for various periods, and spiramycin 2 g daily for two months. Spiramycin may also be used on an alternate-day basis with cotrimoxazole four to six tablets daily.

Selected Readings

Andreev, VC, Angelov, N, Zlatkov, NB: Skin manifestations in toxoplasmosis. *Arch Dermatol* 1969; 100:196.

Binazzi, M: Patologia dermatologica e toxoplasmos: *Ann Ital Dermatol Clin Sper* 1980; 34:369.

Binazzi, M, Papini, M: Cutaneous toxoplasmosis. *Int J Dermatol* 1980; 19:332.

Ippolito, F: Simposio sulla toxoplasmosi. *Bull Int Dermatol S Gall* 1981; 9:1.

Pollock, JL: Toxoplasmosis appearing to be dermatomyositis. *Arch Dermatol* 1979; 115:736.

Toxoplasmosis. *Br Med J* 1981; 282:249.

CHAPTER 23

Onchocerciasis

Onchocerciasis, also known as onchocercosis, caused by a filarial nematode, is probably better known to the lay public by the more graphic name *river blindness*. It is endemic in many areas throughout the sub-Saharan parts of Africa from Nigeria to Tanzania and from Angola to Eritrea; in the Americas, it is most often found in Mexico, Venezuela, and Colombia. Rather surprisingly, there is small focus in the Yemen, but it seems to be unknown in the rest of Asia.

The disease can occur at any age, and over 40 million people are known to be affected, of whom at least 1 percent are now blind. Patients usually live in areas where rapidly running, shallow streams are the preferred breeding sites of the black flies that are the intermediate hosts of the infection and that all belong to the family Simuliidae. These flies need highly oxygenated water in which to breed. Although various members of the family live in different places, the disease is epidemic only in riverine areas. One of the African flies, *Simulium damnosum,* has been known to fly up to 300 kilometers for breeding purposes and so is easily able to extend disease to new areas. In South America, the areas of highest endemicity are usually some 1,000 meters above sea-level, especially in coffee plantations, but different breeding habits of another intermediate host ensure that in Venezuela mainly the coastal regions are affected.

In those parts of Africa where new dams have been built for hydroelectric schemes, spread of water often provides new sites for the Simuliidae to breed and so permits extension of river blindness to previously unaffected populations. Some of the most fertile valleys in Africa have been completely abandoned by the population because of the high incidence of the disease—sometimes as many as 30 percent have impaired vision and more than 5 percent are blind. The World Health Organization reported in 1966 that in some villages in Upper Volta more than 25 percent of the population were totally blind.

Etiology

Onchocerca volvulus is a threadlike filarial worm, the male about 5 cm long and the female anything up to 50 cm. Although some of them live independently in the skin, most of them spend their adult lives clustered in groups being slowly surrounded by a fibrous and inflammatory reaction that produces firm dermal nodules up to 5 cm in diameter known as onchocercomata. The adults cause relatively little trouble; the unpleasant features of the disease are entirely due to the microfilariae produced by the adult female worm. They exist in enormous numbers in the dermis, but the life cycle cannot continue unless they are removed from the skin by one of the Simuliidae that bites an infected host and ingests the microfilariae along with the rest of its meal. The female fly bites viciously during the daytime. These flies do not enter houses and curiously are not much danger to anyone sleeping indoors.

It is in these intermediate hosts that the *O. volvulus* undergoes the normal adventures of the filarial family. Piercing the stomach wall, they move to the thoracic muscles, when, after a series of ecdyses have permitted them to become infective, they proceed to the fly's proboscis and are returned to the main host by the bites of the fly. From there they emigrate along the lympatics into the deeper parts of the skin. About a year later they reach adulthood, start to breed, and more microfilariae are added to the dermal store in which they live for up to 3 years. The adult worms have been known to live for 12 to 15 years, producing waves of microfilariae, but finally they too die off. If the patient has had no further bites from an infected fly the disease will very slowly have reached a natural cure; by then the clinical features will be well established.

Onchocerca volvulus is one of the few filariae that has been known to traverse the placenta. In endemic areas, where most of the population is continually reinfected by repeated bites, it has been said that as many as 5 percent of the children are actually born with the disease.

Clinical Features

In a fully established case, both skin and eyes are majorly infected.

Skin Changes

Starting with an itching that is later associated with erythema, onchodermatitis shows numerous small papules often confined in the first instance to a single area on the trunk or to a single limb. These have at times been mistaken for scabies. Later, large parts of the skin become lichenified (Figure 23-1), and

FIGURE 23-1 Lichenified lesions with scaling and depigmentation. (Courtesy Anezi Okoro, M.D., Enugu, Nigeria.)

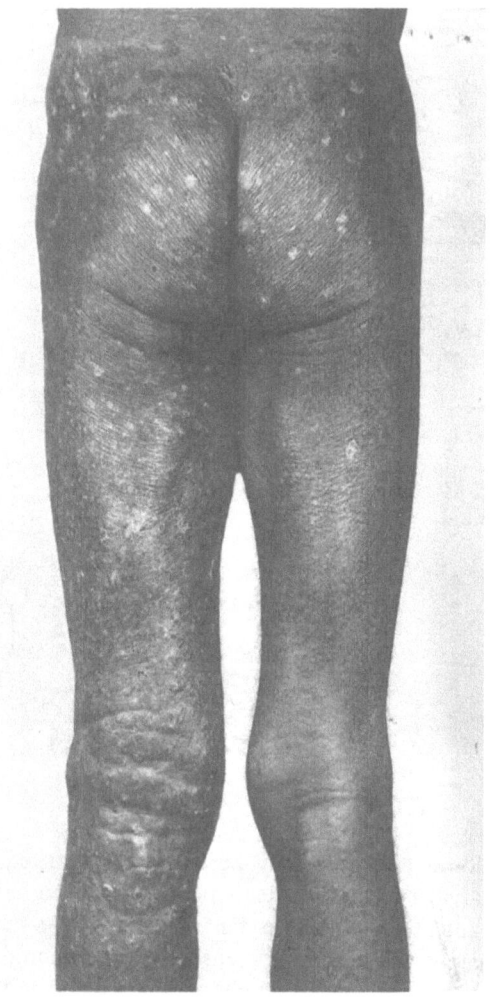

destruction of elastic tissue leads to atrophy and the production of a lax. wrinkled skin, which, if it affects the face, gives a permanently aged appearance.

Further changes in the skin vary in different parts of the world. In the American form of the disease, onchocercomata appear most frequently around the head and neck, perhaps because the *Simulium ochraceum* (the only member of the Simuliidae that is not black) bites mainly this part of the body. In these countries, gross skin changes occur less frequently than in Africa, but sometimes pseudoerysipelas may occur on the face (erysipela de la costa (Figure 23-2). When the lesions lose elasticity and ultimately atrophy, they may take on a form of leonine facies (mal morado).

In the African type of disease, skin changes of the lower limbs, scrotum, and

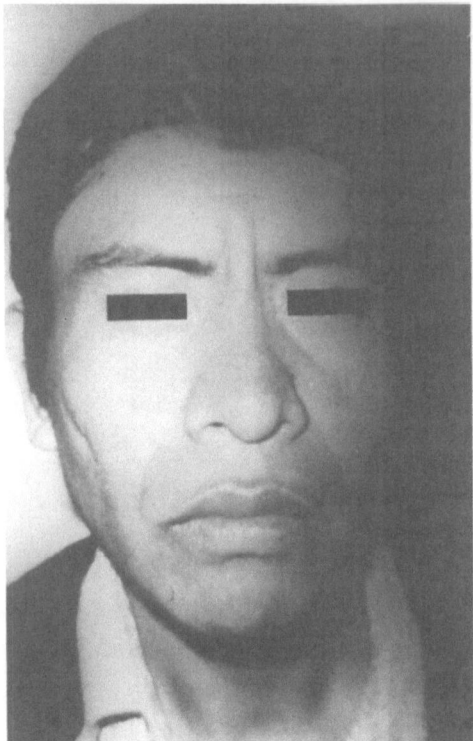

FIGURE 23-2   Dermatitis on face
known as erysipela de la costa.
(Courtesy Arturo Tapia, M.D.,
Panama City, Panama.)

lower abdomen may be extremely marked. The associated onchocercomata
appear most often near the iliac crest; perhaps because the *S. damnosum* usually attacks the lower half of the body. As the years go by, residents in endemic
areas will have an increasingly large microfilarial load, which will cause more
and more severe skin changes. Destruction of the skin's elasticity causes baggy
saccular extensions of the skin, festooning the groins and known as hanging
skin. The more severely affected areas often become achromic. This depigmentation is not necessarily persistent. Often the color returns (as it may do in
vitiligo) by extension of pigment from the pilosebaceous follicles. The outward
spread of the scattered brown spots in a white background is sometimes called
leopard skin.

Onchocercomata are usually rubbery, but after the death of the resident
worms a sterile abscess may form, which can be recognized by the development
of fluctuation in a previously solid nodule.

Lymphadenitis is sometimes found in the hanging skin, while in other
patients, inguinal or femoral hernias, hydroceles, and scrotal enlargment may
develop. Elephantiasis of the scrotum and limbs has been reported from some
parts of Africa and South America, but in other parts it is rare or nonexistent.

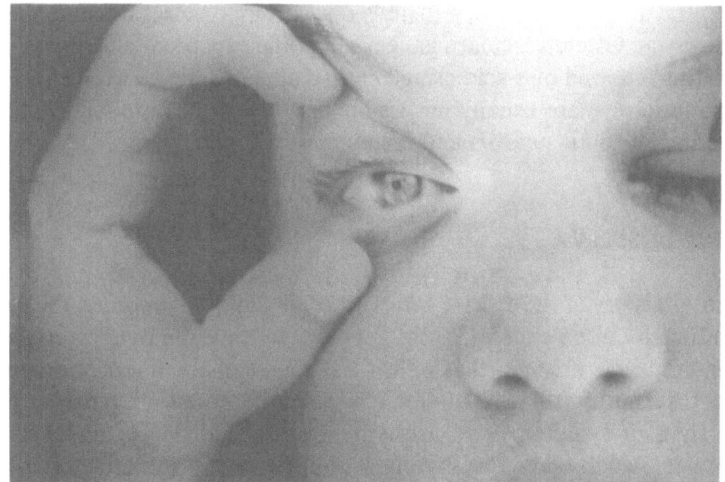

a

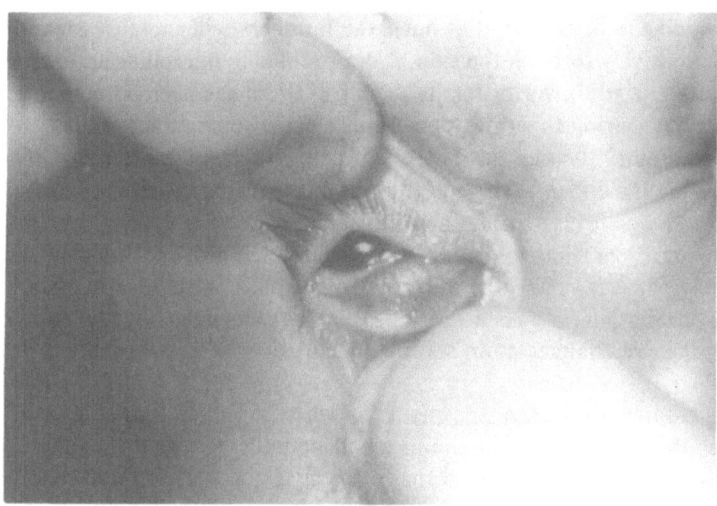

b

FIGURE 23-3a,b   Infected eyelids leading to blindness. (Courtesy Arturo Tapia, M.D., Panama City, Panama.)

Eye Changes

The most disastrous aspects of this disease result from invasion of the eye by microfilariae (Figure 23-3). This most probably occurs by extension from infected eyelids, as blood-borne spread is unusual. Microfilariae of the *O. volvulus*, unlike those of other filariae (*Wuchereria bancrofti, Brugia malayi*, etc.), do not seem to like living in the bloodstream.

When the microfilariae die, a toxin is released that causes direct damage to adjacent tissue. Often, vascular changes affect the eye, producing first a punctate keratitis followed by a sclerosing keratitis and an anterior uveitis. Changes in the posterior eye are usually not visible because of the anterior uveitis, but they can include optic neuritis and finally optic atrophy.

Natural History

The natural history of the disease varies according to whether or not the patient lives continually in an endemic area. People who leave the area after a single infection will show changes that reflect the course of the life of the parasite. For 12 to 18 months after a first infection, while the worms are reaching maturity, no signs or symptoms will appear. After the female begins to produce microfilariae, which enter the skin, an initial itching in the affected areas is followed by the appearance of pruritic papules sometimes called craw. The adult worms continue to produce more microfilariae, and for two or three years (after which the first wave dies out), the numbers will increase steadily and spread extensively through the skin. After producing microfilariae for some 12 to 15 years, the adult worms finally die off. If there has been no reinfection the disease stops. During this time, one or more onchocercomata are likely to have developed around the worms. These will help to focus the attention of physicians outside the endemic sites on the possibility of the disease.

The more severe classical lesions are seen in patients who have been infected on many occasions: lichenification, pigmentary changes, and hanging skin are found only when regular superinfection by infected Simuliidae compound the number of microfilariae. As a result of this, the skin signs become more exaggerated, the eye changes more severe, and the disease has no chance of dying out.

At the same time, the enormous increases of microfilariae in the skin increases the probability that the flies will be infected whenever they bite, so there will be a greater likelihood that every fly's bite will be infective.

Differential Diagnosis

In the early stage of the disease, particularly in people who have returned home after a visit to the tropics, onchodermatitis may be confused with scabies or pyoderma, while later lichen simplex chronicus, vitiligo, or cutis laxis may all be misdiagnosed at some time or other. Even lepromatous leprosy may be suspected if the patients develop mal morado.

Onchocercomata are usually easy to recognize. If there are no other signs and symptoms, they may be mistaken for a fibroma or a lipoma. A form of hanging skin may also be seen in pseudoxanthoma elasticum.

A combination of these signs, especially when associated with eye changes, makes the diagnosis hard to miss.

Investigations

When the diagnosis is suspected, a search for microfilariae is essential. The skin snip (see Appendix one) easily demonstrates the highly motile microfilariae, but if no microscope is available. another technique may be used to prove their presence. It is the Mazzotti test, in which 50 mg of diethylcarbamazine is given by mouth. Within six hours, a sharp increase in pruritis is associated with the rapid development of small new papules.

Recognition of microfilariae in the anterior chamber of the eye can be helped by an ophthalmoscopic or slit-lamp examination. When the eye has been long blind, these organisms are no longer detectable.

A white blood count will invariably show a high eosinophilia. Such a finding simply suggests the presence of a parasite and can be no more specific, but the *absence* of eosinophilia in a patient suspected of having the disease will be evidence against such a diagnosis.

Immunologic tests are of little value because they not only cross-react with other filarial infections, but almost everybody in an endemic area will show a positive reaction. If a microfilarial antigen from *O. volvulus* is available, a positive reaction may be diagnostically helpful in an early case in someone living in a nonendemic area (see Appendix two).

Treatment

As for other filarial diseases, diethylcarbamazine is the drug of choice. Two 4 mg/kg doses three times a day for 14 days is highly effective against the microfilariae, but is not sufficient to kill the adult worms. Repeated courses are necessary to cover the remorseless production of fresh waves of microfilariae from adult females loose in the skin or living in the onchocercomata.

As the destruction of intraocular microfilariae may lead to a severe reaction in the eye, it is suggested that the first course should start slowly.

Day 1	50 mg once (in effect this is a Mazzotti test)
Day 2	50 mg twice
Day 3	50 mg three times
Day 4	100 mg three times
Days 5–14	250 mg three times daily

Even if an ocular reaction is not expected, mydriatics and steroid eyedrops should always be available.

As an alternative treatment, suramin is more active against the adult worms, but it has to be administered with care. Its dosage and limitations are considered on page 198.

Most patients do not have many onchocercomata. and, as they are not firmly attached to adjacent tissue their surgical shelling-out is a practical possibility. If the majority of adult worms can be removed in a single operation there will be a better chance of rapid cure. In some areas, mass "nodulectomy" has been followed by a reduction in the incidence of new cases.

Prevention

Mass treatment of communities must be done with great care and suitable medical back-up, as some people submitted to such prophylaxis may already be infected, and a severe reaction to diethylcarbamazine can cause severe ophthalmic complications.

Destruction of the Simuliidae has been attempted by spraying DDT from an aircraft over the resting places of *S. damnosum*. There has so far been no evidence of DDT resistance.

Selected Readings

Buck, AA: *Onchocerciasis: Symptomatology, Pathology, Diagnosis.* Geneva, WHO, 1974.

Connor, DH: Current concepts in parasitology: Onchocerciasis. *N Engl J Med* 1978; 298:379.

Nelson, GS: Onchocerciasis. *Adv Parasitol* 1970; 8:173.

Ree, GH: Onchocerciasis treated with diethylcarbamazine. *Br J Dermatol* 1977; 97:551.

Somorin, AO: Onchocerciasis. *Int J Dermatol* 1983; 22:182.

CHAPTER 24

Filariasis

Newcomers to the problems caused by filariae may be excused if they find the nomènclature more than usually confusing, as not all the diseases caused by these nematodes are called filariasis. A filarial worm known as *Onchocerca volvulus* causes onchocerciasis and the Loa loa filaria produces loiasis. The condition that is normally known as filariasis is caused by representatives from the genus *Wuchereria* and from the genus *Brugia* (Brug called them *Wuchereria*, but the name was changed in his honor). Only one form of *Wuchereria* is known *(Wuchereria bancrofti)*. Although many forms of *Brugia* have been recognized, most of them are not pathogenic, and only *B. malayi* and *B. timori* cause natural infection in humans.

W. bancrofti produces Bancroftian filariasis and is found most often in the tropical areas of Africa, Asia, and Oceania. It was once epidemic in some parts of the United States but is found now only in the Caribbean and nearby parts of Central and South America.

Malayan filariasis, caused by *B. malayi*, occurs in the coastal areas of Southeast Asia, spreading north to Japan. It has only recently disappeared from north Australia. Filariasis also occurs in certain Pacific Islands, but parasitologists do not agree as to whether it is caused by *W. bancrofti* or a different organism called *W. pacifica*. The disease can affect anyone in the endemic areas at any time; sex, age, and race are no bar to a sting from an infected mosquito.

Etiology

The female *W. bancrofti* is up to 10 cm long, the male about half that size. These white, threadlike worms are usually found in lymphatic vessels and lymph nodes, the sexes being coiled together and separable only with difficulty.

B. malayi is practically indistinguishable from *W. bancrofti;* the *B. malayi* females seem identical, but perhaps are somewhat shorter, and the difference between the microfilariae is rather more marked. Differentiation is of little use to a clinician however, treatment is the same for both infections.

The final host of these filariae is humans, in whom they mate in the connective tissue and lymphatics. the female laying eggs in which larvae have already formed. To develop further, the microfilariae must enter the bloodstream, where they are taken up by certain types of mosquito. Many species of *Culex, Aedes,* and *Anopheles* have been shown at various times and in various places to serve as the intermediate host.

Within a few hours of ingestion, the microfilariae bore their way out of the stomach and migrate into the thoracic muscle, where following two ecdyses, they turn into an infective form that then moves to the mosquito's proboscis, leaving while the mosquito is taking another blood meal. Having returned to their final host, they proceed to a suitable situation in a lymphatic vessel (especially the lymph nodes, the testis, and the spermatic cord), where they may live for a year or more. Toward the end of this time they mature, and the cycle recommences.

The *B. malayi* undergoes an essentially similar cycle, but it is known that on occasion it may invade cats and monkeys as reservoir hosts.

For reasons that are unknown, after the eggs have been laid in humans the microfilariae only appear in the bloodstream at specific times; *W. bancrofti* is detectable between 10 P.M. and 2 A.M., except in the Polynesian islands, where they are usually found in the blood in the daytime. *B. malayi* may show periodicity (around midnight), but sometimes it is subperiodic and appears in the evening between 6 and 8 P.M.

Clinical Features

In the early days of infection, an acute inflammatory response may develop, with fever and malaise. Later, orchitis or epididymitis appear if the genitalia are involved (usually in Bancroftian filariasis), while lymphadenitis and lymphangitis of the lower limb is more often seen in Malayan infection. Not infrequently, an urticarial eruption occurs in association with eosinophilia.

Slowly, enlarged lymph nodes, lymphedema, or hydrocele may develop, and there may be repeated attacks of lymphangitis caused by dying worms. As the condition becomes more fully established, increasing lymphedema is followed by elephantiasis (Figure 4-1), and the lower limb may ultimately produce a verrucose hyperplasia known as mossy foot.

Natural History

Most infected individuals never have any signs or symptoms. Sometimes the disease is recognized only by accidental detection of a microfilaremia. The development of pathologic changes in the lymphatic system only occurs in a

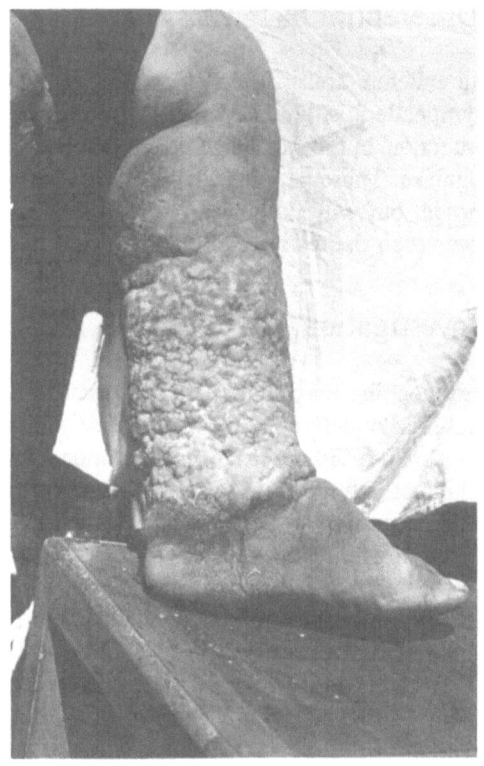

FIGURE 24-1 Long term infestation results and fibrosis, verrucous formation, and elephantiasis. (Courtesy Mohsen Soliman, M.D., Cairo, Egypt.)

small percentage of hosts, probably because of an immunologic reaction to infection.

Lymphadenitis and lymphedema of the scrotum or limb, usually unilateral, may not appear until the infection has been present for many years. Blockage causes transudation of lymph into the connective tissue, and a subsequent proliferation of fibrous tissue results in elephantiasis. The swelling, which may be enormous, is usually smooth. Only rarely does mossy foot complicate the picture.

Other lymphatic complications may be seen: chyluria, chyloceles (in the scrotum), or even chylothorax.

Tropical Eosinophyllic Lung

Sometimes patients may complain of cough and malaise and are found to have a diffuse pulmonary infiltration, as well as a very high eosinophilia. It is believed that many of these patients are suffering from an unrecognized filariasis, but in many cases it is not possible to confirm the presence of microfilariae.

Differential Diagnosis

In endemic areas, fevers, malaise, insomnia, fatigue, urticaria, lymphangitis, lymphadenitis, lymphedema, hydrocele, or chyluria may all indicate a filarial infection, but if the filaria are not detected such cases may easily remain unrecognized. Those patients with a filarial elephantiasis are more likely to be diagnosed, but only if the search for microfilaria is done at a suitable time, and even then the tests are often negative if the disease is of long standing.

Investigation

Eosinophilia may suggest that a parasite is present, but it is only in tropical pulmonary eosinophilia that extremely high percentages have been recorded (up to 70 or 80 percent). The common forms of filariasis stimulate an eosinophilia of only 10 to 15 percent which is of no specific diagnostic help.

Recognition of the organisms in the blood is the most helpful finding. Thick blood films may be stained with Giemsa stain, but this is not really necessary as the microfilariae may be detected with a hand lens if the smear is made with infected blood. By the time lymphedema and elephantiasis have appeared, microfilaremia is no longer dependable.

In such cases it may be possible to recognize parts of the worm in a biopsy from an inguinal lymph node or some other infected tissue, but usually the section only shows evidence of chronic infection with epithelioid cells, giant cells, and tissue eosinophilia, and no specific diagnosis can be made.

A skin test made from the dog heartworm *Dirofilaria immitis* has given variable results. Similar tests made from *W. bancrofti* and *B. malayi* can cross-react with intestinal helminths and cannot be relied on as a diagnostic aid.

Treatment

Most of the symptoms that cause a patient to be diagnosed as having filariasis are not helped by successful antifilarial treatment. Diethylcarbamazine (4 to 6 mg/kg) daily for 14 days is highly effective against the microfilariae, but destruction of the adults will require a further two to three weeks. Mebendazole 1 g twice daily for 28 days is sometimes used instead.

If diethylcarbamazine is not successful, suramin may be given against the adult worms. It is nephrotoxic and should not be used by people with albumin or casts in their urine. Other patients can be given suramin intravenously (1 g in 10 ml water) once a week for eight weeks, but only if they do not respond adversely to a test dose of 200 mg.

In some cases, repeated febrile episodes will require systemic corticosteroids for several weeks, while any secondary infection that develops will need appropriate antibiotics.

Local treatment of lymphedema may be helpful; the swelling can be reduced by firmly binding a previously elevated limb, starting from the foot and including the whole leg. Treatment must be maintained for several weeks and preferably a two-way stretch elastic bandage should be used (such as Elastoplast).

Prevention

In most parts of the world, mass treatment can be expected to eradicate filariasis, as there is usually no other reservoir host but humans. Unfortunately, patient acceptance is not good because the severe reactions that are sometimes produced by diethylcarbamazine often dissuade many people from accepting medication. Partial success has been obtained in some areas by adding the medication to cooking salt.

The other approach to prevention is to undertake mass control of the mosquito vectors by suitable techniques. Dieidrin and DDT sprays may be used against those *Anopheles* that are not resistant. Careful campaigns to instigate village control of *Aedes* breeding sites within 100 meters of the village will diminish the possibilities of *Aedes* transmission because of its short flight range.

Selected Readings

Joe, LK: Occult filariasis: Its relationship with tropical pulmonary eosinophilia. *Am J Trop Med Hyg* 1962; 11:646.

Maegraith, B: *Adams and Maegraith: Clinical Tropical Diseases*. London, Blackwell Scientific, 1980, pp 64–82.

Nelson GS: Current concepts in parasitology: Filariasis. *N Engl J Med* 1979; 300:1136.

Neva, FA, Ottesen, EA: Tropical (filarial) eosinophilia. *N Engl J Med* 1978; 298:1129.

Richards, RN: Verrucous and elephantoid lymphedema. *Int J Dermatol* 1981; 20:177.

CHAPTER 25

Dracunculosis

Dracunculosis, also known as dracontiasis, dracunculiasis, or guinea-worm disease, is one of the oldest known diseases, accounts having been found in Egyptian as well as in early Greek and Roman writings. It has been suggested that the guinea worm was the "fiery serpent" that chased the Israelites during their wanderings around the Red Sea. It is also believed that the physician's symbol, the caduceus, which has a worm around a stick, may well have originated as a depiction of the guinea worm.

The disease exists mainly in the drier parts of the tropics and subtropics of Africa, the Indian subcontinent, and the Middle East. It also appears in certain parts of the Caribbean and South America.

Etiology

The disease is caused by the *Dracunculus medinensis,* which reaches sexual maturity in its final host, humans. Having mated, the male dies and the female migrates slowly to the lower part of the leg, where it moves to the surface and apparently secretes a toxin that causes a blister to develop. This breaks down when the leg is cooled with water, the worm lying under this erosion discharges millions of larvae by repeated contractions of the uterus, which takes up most of its body. The female worm can be more than 60 cm long but is only 2 to 3 mm in diameter.

After exposure to water, the embryo larvae uncurl and become active. They only survive a few days in clear water but last for up to two to three months in muddy water or moist soil. If the soil dries up completely, the larvae will become active again when more water arrives. In this water certain small crustacea of the genus *Cyclops* are attracted by the movement of the larvae and ingest thousands of them. Within a few weeks the larvae become infective.

The final host (humans or certain animals) swallows these crustacea by drinking contaminated water. In the host's alimentary tract, the *Cyclops* is destroyed, releasing larvae that migrate through the gastrointestinal mucosa into surrounding tissue. There, the process of maturation takes up to a year before the cycle starts again.

Clinical Features

During the phase of maturation, there is little if any evidence that the patient is infected. When the traveling female arrives in the leg (occasonally it can be found in the scrotum or elsewhere), the skin begins to itch, and a red papule develops rapidly into a blister that may be five or more centimeters in diameter. The base is indurated and edematous. The bulla soon erodes, leaving an ulcer with a central punctum through which the worm protrudes when provoked by immersion in water that is below body temperature. The uterus is extruded through the punctum and discharges a cloudy larvae-containing fluid into the water or over the ulcer. When the blister begins to appear, there may be an associated systemic reaction—general malaise, diarrhea, vomiting—probably in reaction to the toxin that enables the worm to create a bulla.

Natural History

The first clinical evidence that a person has dracunculosis is usually the appearance of a papule on the lower portion of the leg that rapidly develops into a bulla. It may at that time be possible to palpate the worm lying in the subcutaneous tissue (Figure 25-1).

It is not unknown for the worm to become damaged during its migration, particularly when it has arrived in the subcutaneous tissue but has not yet caused a blister. If this happens, cellulitis or even a sterile abscess may develop, which, if it occurs near a joint, may cause effusion or arthritis. It has been reported that some patients develop a fibrosis constricting the tendons of the legs.

On other occasions, secondary infection of the ulcerated bulla will produce a cellulitis around the affected part. When the worm is superficial enough to be palpated, it can also be visible (especially if the scrotum is involved), and there may be a superficial resemblance to larva migrans.

Differential Diagnosis

The classic presentation of a single large blister with an erythematous base on the lower part of the leg or the foot can rarely be mistaken for anything else, particularly if the limb is put into a bucket of cold water. There is a consequent cloudy discharge of innumerable larvae.

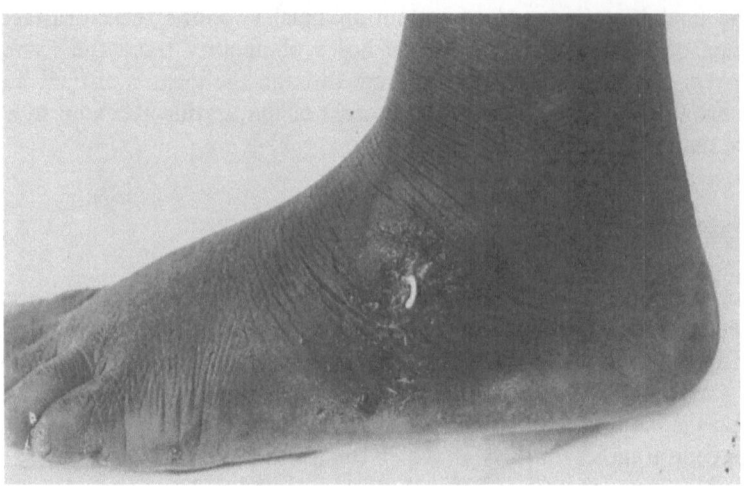

FIGURE 25-1   The guinea worm exuding from the ankle, which is indurated and edematous. (Courtesy Anezi Okoro, M.D., Enugu, Nigeria.)

There is much more of a diagnostic problem if the classical lesion has not
yet developed and a subcutaneous abscess appears elsewhere. Evacuation of the
pus will usually show that necrosis has been associated with the presence of a
dead guinea worm. If a joint (knee or ankle) is affected, it may be wrongly
taken for rheumatism, traumatic synovitis, or even sciatica, but these relatively
unusual presentations can be detected by an x-ray of the area, which usually
shows a calcified worm in the tissue.

The superficial resemblance to larva migrans does not usually cause diagnostic problems, as the history is not the same. In larva migrans, no worm can
be felt in the skin.

Sometimes the bulla is not seen and the patient seeks attention for an
infected ulcer, which may be confused with anything from pyoderma to a
Buruli ulcer. The palpation of the worm will show the true diagnosis.

Investigations

Up to 15 percent eosinophila may be found in many cases. The diagnosis cannot be based on this finding alone, but it may be of help in confirming suspi-
cions based on other symptoms.

Live, unruptured worms in the deeper tissues usually cannot be detected,
but if the worm dies, they may become calcified and so demonstrable on x-ray.
More often, however, dead worms are simply absorbed.

It is rarely necessary to biopsy a skin lesion. If this is done, evidence will be found of acute or chronic infection, including giant cells, epithelioid cells, and some eosinophils. Some part of a degenerating worm may also be present.

Some workers have used an intradermal test with an antigen made from the dried powdered worm, but these investigations have not found general acceptance.

Treatment

Removal of the worm is obviously the best way to correct the situation and the traditional folk practice, still used in many areas, is to attach the protruding worm to a stick or a match and slowly to wind it out 2 to 3 cm at a time until the whole worm has been removed. Unfortunately, not only may the worm be torn by an enthusiastic operator but sometimes the winding will push eggs back into the worm until it bursts. In either case, the subsequent painful, angry inflammation of the subcutaneous tissue can become secondarily infected and often needs to be treated with systemic antibiotics.

It is better to treat the condition by systemic therapy; metronidazole can be given (25 mg/kg daily for ten days). Thiabendazole is equally effective but its unpleasant side effects make it less acceptable.

Urticarial elements are sometimes seen. They respond well to antihistamines provided the dracunculus is suppressed at the same time. Surgically oriented doctors have sometimes preferred to dissect the worm out, but this is not easy if, as may happen, several worms are present at the same time.

Prevention

The disease usually occurs in areas where the same sources are used for washing and drinking. It will never be eliminated until infected individuals stop contaminating their water supply. Provision of good clean piped water is therefore a prime necessity. If this is not possible, attempts have to be made to destroy the secondary host (the *Cyclops*) by suitable treatment of water. They can be killed by heating the water before it is drunk (a difficult solution in many parts of the world) or the source can be treated by a molluscicide such as Temephos, one part per million. Wells can also be treated by perchloron, a bleaching powder substitute. It is claimed that if the barbel fish, which feeds voraciously on the *Cyclops,* is introduced into the water supply, guinea-worm disease disappears from the neighborhood.

If such public health precautions are not carried out, the population of infected areas is liable to be affected many times, as there is no immunologic protection against the worms or their larvae.

Selected Readings

After small-pox, guinea worm?, editorial. *Lancet* 1983; 1:161.
Kale, OO: Clinical evaluation of drugs for dracontiasis. *Trop Doct* 1977; 7:15.
Muller, R: Dracunculus and dracunculiasis. *Ad Parasitol* 1971; 9:73.
Muller, R: Guinea worm disease: Epidemiology, control and treatment. *Bull WHO;* 1979; 57:683.

CHAPTER 26

Schistosomiasis

Ten percent of the world's population is infected with schistosomiasis, which has been known in Egypt for 4,000 years. Often called bilharzia, it is a major cause of ill health in the tropics and subtropical regions. In 1851, Dr. T. Bilharz first described the adult form of schistosomal helminths, or flatworms, living in the portal veins of humans, but not until early in the twentieth century was it recognized that different forms of watersnails act as intermediate hosts for the different forms of schistosomiasis. Three of these worms can affect humans: *Schistosoma haematobium,* which is prevalent in Africa and the Middle East, *S. mansoni,* which occurs both in Africa and South America, and *S. japonicum,* which is found in the Far East. In certain parts of Africa not only do *S. haematobium* and *S. mansoni* exist together, but it is not unknown, particularly in the Sudan and in upper Egypt, for patients to be affected by both parasites at once.

As the snails that are the intermediate hosts for these nematodes prefer to live in fresh water, a recent change in the method of irrigation in Egypt and elsewhere has encouraged spread of the disease. Previously, the basin method of irrigation (depending on the rise and fall of the water level in the rivers) did not favor these snails. Since the building of the Aswan Dam, however, the irrigation has become perennial, and the hosts of both *S. mansoni* and *S. haematobium* have thrived and extended through much of the Nile Valley. The snails prefer the water to be alkaline and to contain calcium; both these needs are fulfilled in many parts of South America, but as they do not like cold water. Bilharzia cannot be acquired outside the tropics or at an altitude of much more than 1,500 meters.

Etiology

Only three species of *Schistosoma* cause serious disease. In *S. haematobium* humans are the main reservoir and only rarely has this fluke been found in other animals. This is the organism that causes vesical or urinary bilharzia. *S. mansoni* has been found in other primates as well as in humans and is the cause of intestinal bilharzia. *S. japonicum* is limited to the Far East and affects dogs, cats, rats, mice, cattle, buffalo, pigs, and many other animals besides humans. It has been estimated that in the Phillipines some 25 percent of schistosomiasis is caused by contamination of water supplies by such animals. In China, rats living on the river banks are responsible for the spread of the disease and the use of human feces for fertilizer is an additional public health hazard.

All of these organisms have essentially the same life cycle. Cercerial larvae from many other schistosomes are known to penetrate the skin of human beings who are unwise enough to put themselves or their lower limbs into infected water but most of these larvae cannot mature in humans and soon die off.

The cerceria from the three pathogens do not die but move via the lymphatics into the bloodstream and travel through the heart and lungs into the hepatic portal vessels, in which they mature. Some 100 to 500 μ in length, the leaflike male rolls up to form a tube that encloses a cylindrical female. Having paired, they migrate to the veins of their choice, *S. haematobium* going to veins around the bladder while the others prefer to live in the mesenteric vessels. In these sites, they lay many hundreds of eggs each day that penetrate through the walls of the intestine or bladder and ultimately may be found in the urine or feces, along with which they reach the outside world. When the ova enter water, a myracidium is hatched that can live for about 48 hours. The cycle cannot continue unless the myracidium is swallowed by a suitable snail, in which it develops into a tube-shaped "mother" sporocyst from which emerge parthenogenitically numerous "daughter" sporocysts, which produce infective cercarial larvae. These pass out of the respiratory aperture of the snail and reenter water, where, if they encounter their main host, they cast their forked tails, penetrate the skin, and complete the cycle.

Clinical Features

Various dermatologic manifestations accompany different stages of infection and can be divided into three types.

Invasive Schistosomiasis

When the cercerial larvae penetrate the skin for the first time, an inflammatory reaction must be expected (especially to those avian species that penetrate the skin only to die off). A mixture of irritant and allergic manifestations, sometimes called schistosome dermatitis, starts with itching as the cercariae touch the skin. As the water evaporates and penetration is completed, an increased pruritus is associated with macules, papules, and excoriations that soon become pustular and crusted. The dermatitis increases in severity for two or three days and subsides within two weeks. On rare occasions, when these lesions are seen by a physician, they are usually given a nonspecific name such as swimmer's itch. The true diagnosis is made only in retrospect.

Patients who live in endemic areas and are continually being reinfected do not show these early manifestations, having probably acquired an immunity.

Urticarial Schistosomiasis

This too is usually only found in patients who have not previously been infected. Some four to six weeks after cercarial invasion, the flukes mature, and fever, arthralgia, cough, eosinophilia, and lymphadenopathy develop, probably because the sudden appearance of thousands of ova produce an immunologic cross-reaction with antigens that have developed as a reaction to the growing worms. On the skin, red macules, itching papules, urticaria, and even angioneurotic edema can be seen. This reaction is most severe with *S. japonicum*. In Japan, it is called urticarial fever or Katayama disease.

Cutaneous Schistosomiasis

This will develop after the systemic signs of bilharzia begin to appear. Although ova most frequently invade the bladder or the gut, they may be found anywhere in the neighborhood, and in any site they may provoke a slowly growing granuloma. Sometimes these lesions are seen in the skin (especially the perineum and adjoining genital region). A fibrotic papilloma with draining sinuses and fistulae may appear, which in Egypt have been known to extend through the crural folds to affect the labia and clitoris and even cause a pseudoelephantiasis of the vulva (Figure 26-1).

As the infections become more severe, granulations may form around the umbilicus if the flukes have invaded the periumbilical veins (Figure 26-2) and hard, flat papules appear on the chest that later coalesce to form a skin-colored plaque. Later still, a watering-can perineum may result from fistulous connections between the bladder and the skin.

Dermatologic manifestations of schistosomiasis are rarely diagnosed until systemic disease has become recognizable.

Natural History

The first symptom of urinary schistosomiasis recognized by the patient is hematuria, particularly toward the end of micturition. Microscopy of the urinary sediment shows blood cells and the diagnostic ova. As the disease slowly

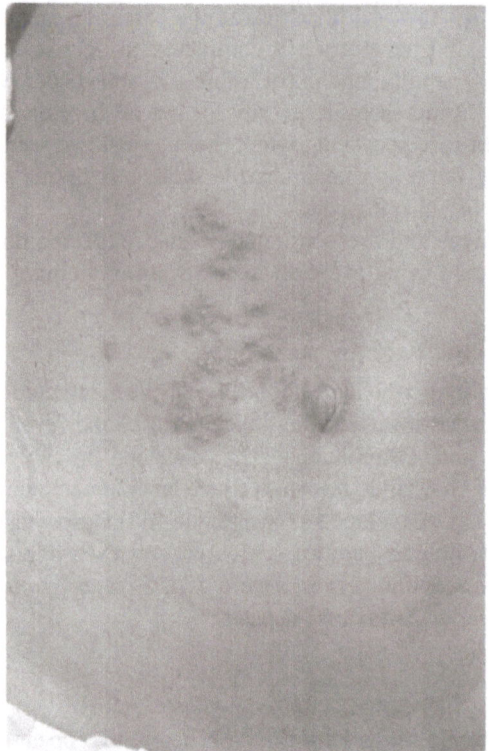

FIGURE 26-1 Papules and fibrosis. (Courtesy Mohsen Soliman, M.D., Cairo, Egypt.)

progresses, cystitis, bladder hypertrophy, hydronephrosis, calculus formation, ureteric obstruction, and urinary fistulae may all develop, and ultimately renal tract infection and uremia may lead to death.

S. mansoni and *S. japonicum* infections start with typhoid-like symptoms—bloody stools and hepato-splenomegaly—but in the early stages ova are not to be found in the feces. As time goes on, acute intestinal complications develop as a result of the ova penetrating the wall of the gut, and dysenteric fever and abdominal pain may last for many months. These symptoms seem to be more prominent in South America than they are in Africa. Later, polyps and papillomata appear in any part of the colon. If they extend to the rectum, soft, friable, granulomatous lesions appearing at the anus can spread to the perineum.

The disease shows little tendency to natural remission. It becomes more and more severe, particularly in patients who are repeatedly infected when fishing, swimming, or bathing in infested water. Anemia, cirrhosis of the liver, uremia, and malignant degeneration in the chronically infected areas may all take their

FIGURE 26-2   Swelling and drain-
ing sinuses in groin. (Courtesy
Mohsen Soliman, M.D., Cairo,
Egypt.)

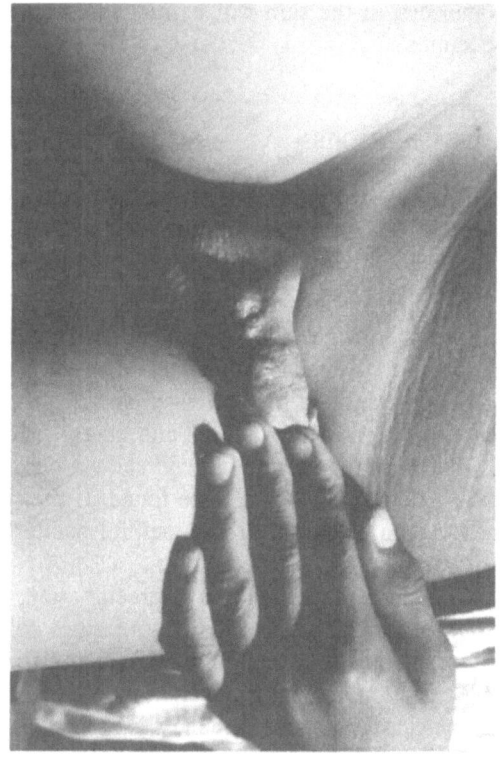

toll unless satisfactory early treatment is available. It must be remembered that
severe symptoms affect only a small portion of the millions of infected people,
and carriers of the disease do not seek medical assistance.

Differential Diagnosis

Invasive schistosomiasis may easily be confused with the cercarial dermatitis
caused by those other schistosomes that do not cause systemic disease, but only
time will tell whether or not a pathogen is involved. If newly infected patients
take their invasive schistosomiasis back to the United States, they may be
thought to have chiggers. Although both scabies and onchocercal dermatitis
may look similar, they have a wider distribution and are not limited to sites
that have been immersed in water.

Urticarial fever may be mistaken for other sorts of toxic erythema or urticaria and even for allergic vasculitis. The granulomatous reactions to schisto-

somal ova in the skin will be diagnosed only if the ova are seen in a biopsy specimen.

Investigations

It is most unlikely that invasive or urticarial disease will ever be diagnosed other than retrospectively, and investigations taken in the early stages of infection are of very little help.

If systemic schistosomiasis is suspected, a search should be made for ova in the stools or urine. They may be differentiated from each other by the position of spines on the shell: *S. haematobium* has a terminal spine at one of the poles of the oval egg, both *S. mansoni* and *S. japonicum* have lateral spines, quite large in the former and small and barely visible in the latter.

Biopsy of the granuloma will show a chronic inflammatory histology, and, with luck, the ova will also be found. If the spines are recognizable, the diagnosis is completed. A further helpful pointer is that shells of *S. mansoni* are acid-fast and the others are not.

Complement-fixation tests, precipitation, and fluorescent antibody techniques are available, but many authorities believe they are of little aid in clinical practice. Intradermal injection of adult worm antigen will produce a positive reaction in almost every inhabitant of endemic areas. It is of more diagnostic significance if the test is positive in a patient living in a nonendemic area who is suspected of having been infected during a visit overseas.

Treatment

In the recent past, different schistosomes responded best to different therapies. It is now recognized that praziquantel, a heterocyclic pyrazino-isoquinoline, is effective against all those forms which affect man, being given as a single dose of 50/mg/kg or two doses of 30 mg/kg at an interval of 12 hours.

If this drug is not available, the treatment of choice against *S. hematobium* is metrifonate which is an organophosphorus compound given in doses of 10 mg/kg every 14 days for 3 doses. The alternative treatment for *S. mansoni* is oxamniquine 20 mg/kg daily for three days. Neither of these drugs is much use against the other types of disease.

Until recently, oral niridazole was used against all the parasites, but occasionally it could cause severe toxic effects (especially in patients with hepatosplenomegaly) and sometimes even caused death from hepatic necrosis. Both this and hycanthone are now rarely used.

It is a wise precaution when treatment has finished to ensure that the ova being excreted are no longer viable (see Appendix one). If myracidia are still found to be hatching from the eggs, a further course of treatment is indicated.

Prevention

Attempts to destroy snails by molluscicides have not been particularly successful. In some communities the introduction of snail-eating ducks to live in the nearby water has been of some help in reducing the incidence of the disease in the neighborhood, but the only real way to ensure the eradication of schistosomiasis is by major changes in public health and personal hygiene. Contaminated urine and feces must be entirely prevented from entering water in which human beings immerse themselves.

Selected Readings

Amer, M: Cutaneous schistosomiasis. *Int J Dermatol* 1982; 21:44.
Bayer, HM: Schistosomiasis. *Int J Dermatol* 1980; 19:168.
Gilles, HM: The treatment of schistosomiasis. *J Microbiolochem* 1981; 7:113.
Jordan, P, Christie, JD, Unrau, GO: Schistosomiasis transmission with particular reference to possible ecological and biological methods of control. *Acta Trop* (Basel) 1980: 37:95.
Pearson, RD, Guerrant, RL: Praziquantel: A major advance in anthelminthil therapy. *Ann Int Med* 1983; 99:195.
Torres, VM: Dermatologic manifestations of schistosomiasis. *Arch Dermatol* 1976; 112:1539.

Other Dermatoses

Part five

Other Dermatoses

CHAPTER 27

Lichen Planus Tropicus

Lichen planus tropicus, also known as lichen planus subtropicus and lichen planus actinicus, is sometimes confused and categorized with actinic reticuloid. It is categorized by annular plaques with minimally raised borders and bluish-brown centers.

Although by definition most of the cases have been reported in tropical areas, there is increased awareness of this disease. It has been found in the United States, Italy, and other nontropical countries. The incidence is unknown, but it does appear to affect patients of all races and both sexes.

It usually begins about the age of 11. Eighty-three percent of the patients are younger than 41, whereas only 38 percent of patients with regular lichen planus are that age.

Whether the disease actually exists is open to speculation. Lichen planus itself was first described by Erasmus Wilson in 1869. Over six decades ago, both John Fordyce in America and Graham Little in the United Kingdom commented on a peculiar type of lichen planus that existed on exposed areas. The disease was codified in 1949 by Dostrovsky and Sagher in Jerusalem, where for 20 years they had followed patients who developed annular pigmented patches, generally on the forehead. Lichen planus tropicus is responsible for 30 to 40 percent of the patients with lichen planus in the tropics. The incidence is slightly higher in women than in men. Some observers have believed that socioeconomic conditions play a role, since lower- to middle-class people are afflicted. Possibly this is due to their excessive exposure to sunlight.

Etiology

The cause of all forms of lichen planus is unknown. Drug reactions and immunologic responses have been postulated for the cause of this papulosquamous disease, but without confirmation. Sun damage in some form precipitates lichen planus tropicus, as evidenced by the lesions appearing on the exposed areas, such as the forehead, scalp, and hands. Lesions are known to lessen during the cold months.

Clinical Features

Pruritic, red, papular lesions can be found on the forehead, cheeks, the dorsal portions of the hands and arms, and extensor surfaces of the legs (Figure 27-1a,b). Sometimes the lesions take on an annular appearance. Lesions that are originally bluish-brown eventually become raised, with a central dell. Sometimes they coalesce and the scaling is minimal (Figure 27-2a,b). The itching is worse in strong sunlight.

The scalp is affected only when the patient has no protective hair. On occasion, lesions can be found on the covered parts of the body (Figure 27-3) and in the oral mucosa. The nails do not show the longitudinal ridging character-

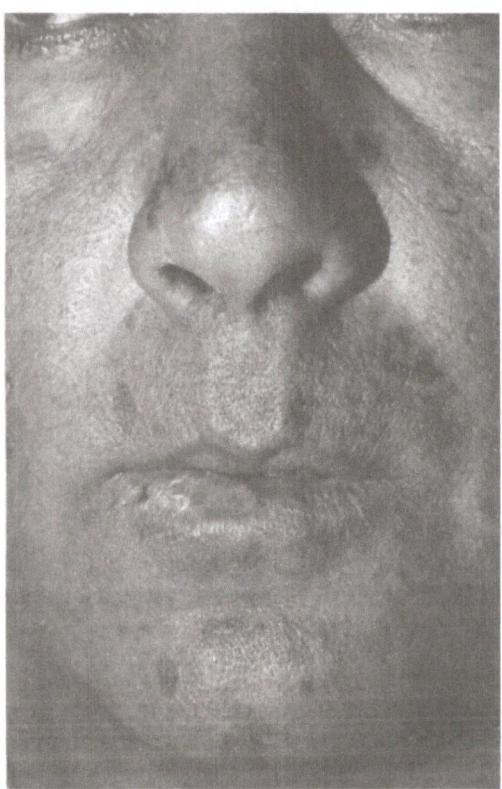

a

FIGURE 27-1a,b Pruritic red (dark areas) papules on the face.

istic of the regular form of lichen planus. In addition, the fine, lacy streaks known as Wickham's striae are generally not present.

Natural History

The course of development is slow. Generally, the disease lasts one to two years but can easily remain for well over a decade.

Differential Diagnosis

The most obvious confusion of this disease occurs with granuloma annulare, but the morphology and distribution would differentiate the two. Similarly, basal cell cancer, discoid lupus erythematosus, elastosis perforans serpiginosa, and porokeratosis of Mibelli head the list of diseases that can mimic lichen planus tropicus. A variety of lichen planus tropicus has been reported from

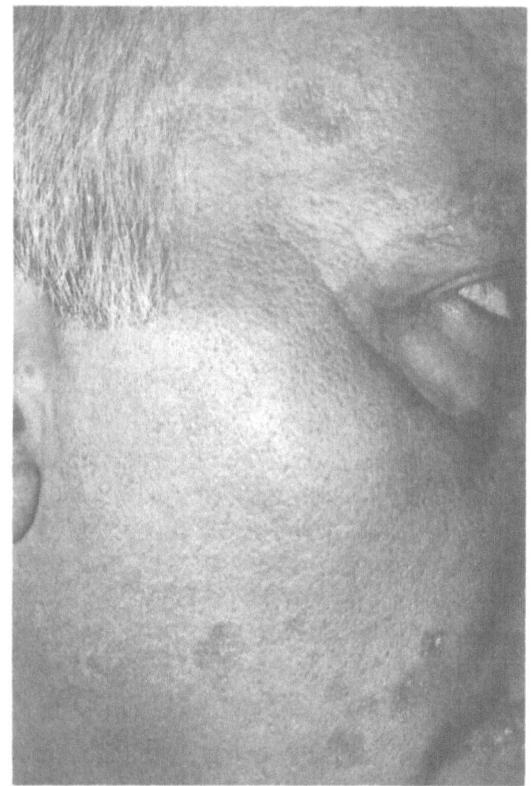

b

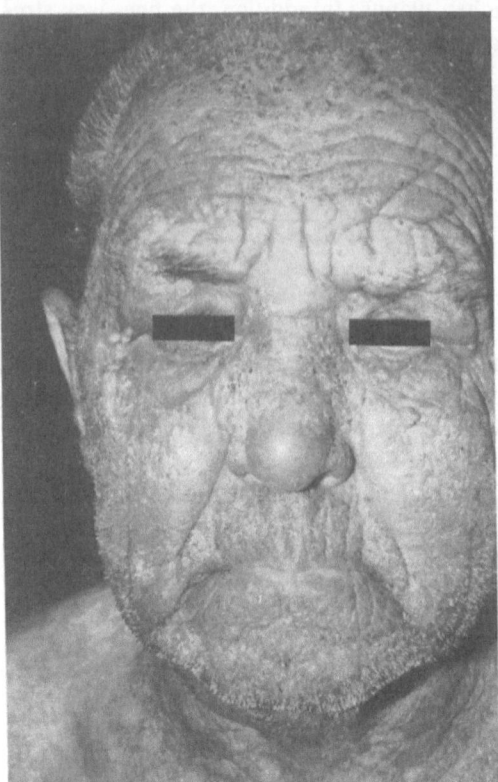

FIGURE 27-2 Actinic reticuloid differs by showing diffuse lichenification and scaling. (All courtesy F. Ayala, M.D., Naples, Italy.)

a

Kenya; Lichenoid melanodermatitis seems to differ by disappearing within eight months. Otherwise, the features are similar.

Investigations

Since the diagnosis is made by inspection, no laboratory tests are necessary, unless a cutaneous biopsy is taken. Routine staining would show hypergranulosis granulosis and thinning and atrophy of the rete ridges, with saw-tooth acanthosis at the edges. Examination of the dermis may show a bandlike infiltrate of lymphocytes next to the epidermis.

Treatment

Like the therapy for lichen planus, the treatment for lichen planus tropicus is not very successful. Topical corticosteroids can reduce the itching, but the disease will generally take its own course.

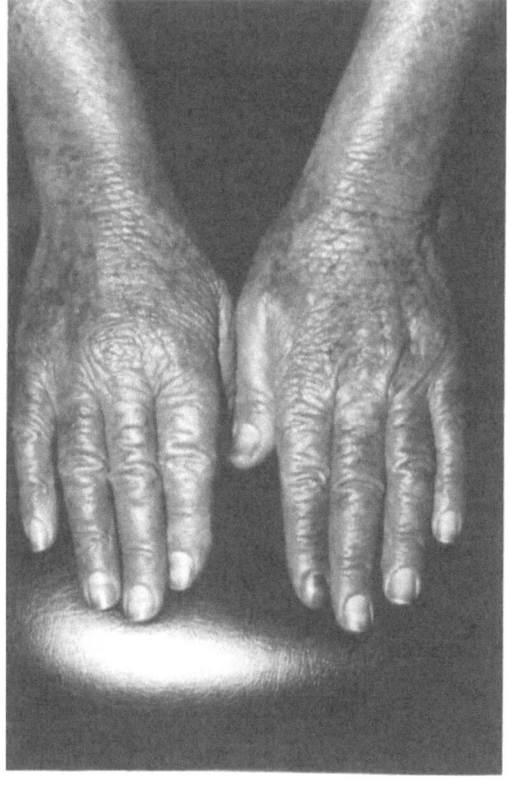

b

FIGURE 27-3   Lichenification, scaling, and red papules in light exposed and nonexposed areas.

With more severe itching, systemic steroids can be considered at 30 to 40 mg a day for a two- to three-week period. Antimalarials, such as chloroquine 500 mg a day for two months, can be considered.

Since the condition appears to be triggered by sunlight, the use of a sunscreen would be indicated.

In any event, the disease generally disappears on its own. Pigmentation can remain as a sequela.

Selected Readings

Dilaimy, M: Lichen planus subtropicus. *Arch Dermatol* 1976; 112:1251.

Dostrovsky, A, Sagher, F: Lichen planus in subtropical countries. *Arch Dermatol Syphilol* 1949; 59:308.

Verhagen, ARHB, Koten, JW: Lichenoid melanodermatitis: A clinicopathologic study of 51 Kenyan patients with so-called tropical lichen planus. *Br J Dermatol* 1979; 101:651.

Zanca, A, Zanca, A: Lichen planus actinicus. *Int J Dermatol* 1978; 17:506.

CHAPTER 28

Dietary Deficiencies

In the middle of 1983, ministers from 36 member countries of the United Nations World Food Council were told that of the 500 million Asians who lived in absolute poverty about 300 million were "endemically undernourished"; that Africa, which 20 years previously had been self-sufficient in food, has replaced Asia as the prinicipal recipient of food supplies, and that in Latin America 70 percent of the rural population shared only 35 percent of the rural income and one in seven was malnourished. Doctors working in western countries should always remember that starvation is the most widespread deficiency disease in the world.

It is a common habit in textbooks to enumerate the vitamins that are necessary to maintain health and to describe individual deficiencies, but the hundreds of millions of people living under starvation circumstances do not complain of such dermatologic niceties as beriberi or pellagra. Famine, war, and natural disaster cause a combination of deficiencies in which skin lesions are the least of the patients' worries, since annually thousands upon thousands of them die of starvation.

It is only in the more affluent countries that the idiosyncracies of dietary cranks, the unbalanced intake of the alcoholic, and the pathetic undernourishment of the solitary aged may manifest specific deficiencies of individual vitamins. Such conditions may be seen in all parts of the world and are not limited to the tropical or subtropical areas.

Kwashiorkor

This name was coined by Cicely Williams in 1933, when she described a constellation of symptoms occurring in children with a low-protein diet whose diet was otherwise balanced, albeit insufficient. The disease may be caused solely by total lack of protein, but it also affects those whose low intake is further reduced by recurrent or persistant diarrhea.

An alternative theory has recently been suggested by workers in the Liverpool School of Tropical Medicine, who noticed that kwashiorkor frequently arises when a child, previously the youngest, is superseded at the breast by an additional younger sibling. Such children not only have a subsequent protein deficiency, but it is suspected that they may also be affected by an aflatoxin produced by a mold that commonly affects food in the hot parts of the world. In the Sudan aflatoxins have been found on food in the markets and even on plates, and in some children very high amounts have been found in the liver. This new theory would explain why some children have been known to die suddenly during the early treatment of the disease—the rapid introduction of a high-protein diet is dangerous to a damaged liver. Not only is it perhaps wiser to introduce the protein slowly to a patient with kwashiorkor but search should be made for a toxoid to stimulate antitoxins to aflatoxin.

Clinical Features

The children are grossly underweight. As the organs of the body fail to develop, there is first an anemia and then a multiplicity of other symptoms and signs, including edema of the legs and face, ascites, and a dry, flaky dyschromia of the skin, sometimes compared to flaky paint. The skin ultimately breaks down, causing necrosis and atrophy. In most patients the hair thins dramatically and changes color, so that the fully established case of kwashiorkor shows an underdeveloped edematous child with startlingly sparse reddish-yellow hair (Figure 28-1a,b).

Associated vitamin deficiencies may be seen, particularly the ocular lesions (Bitot's spots and keratomalacia) caused by diminished vitamin A intake, while intercurrent diseases such as bronchopneumonia or gastrointestinal infections-may cause the condition to end fatally.

Treatment

Patients will respond well to small, frequent feeds of a paste made with skimmed milk powder supplemented with 20 g of sugar per liter and any available edible oil (also 20 g per liter). Vitamin supplements should also be provided.

As the treatment progresses, the edema will disappear in the course of two to three weeks, during which time, rather alarmingly, the child will lose weight. After this interlude, when the diagnosis of marasmus may be mistakenly made, the child improves steadily provided a satisfactorily balanced diet is maintained.

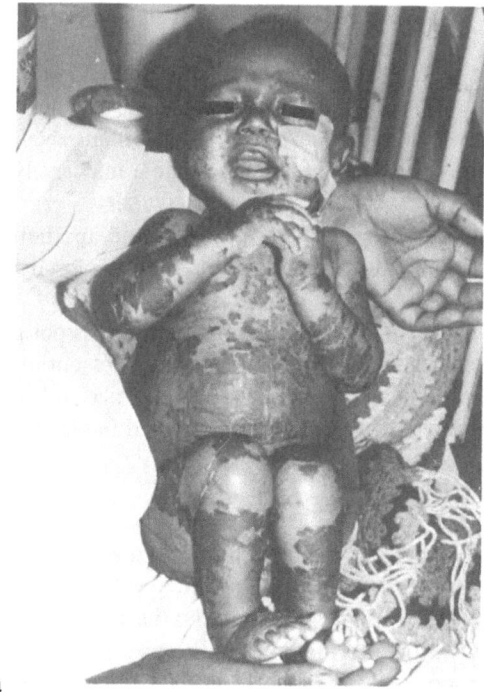

a

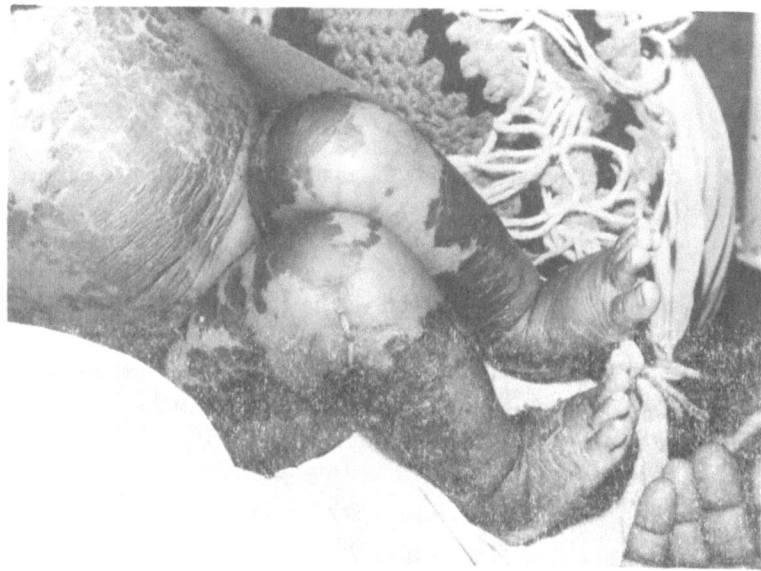

b

FIGURE 28-1a,b   Kwashiorkor: acute disease in a six-month-old child with scaling, desquamation, and hyperpigmentation. (Courtesy J. B. S. Coulter, M.D., Liverpool England.)

Marasmus

Marasmus is caused by a completely inadequate diet and is the most common cause of death from starvation in children. Under famine conditions, these unfortunates are insufficiently breast-fed by undernourished mothers, while infected food or water given as a dietary supplement may easily cause gastrointestinal infections that further reduce the effective diet.

The starving children are grossly underweight and apathetic, with atrophy of all tissues. They do not show the edema or the discolored hair that is seen in kwashiorkor.

It must be ensured that food provided for the family is not given only to the children, as improvement in the diet of the mother is essential if infants are to be breast-fed. Care must also be taken that dried milk and other dehydrated foods are mixed with boiled water and administered in clean feeding bottles.

Vitamin A Deficiency

When it was originally described, the condition known as phrynoderma (see Chapter 29) was attributed to vitamin A deficiency, but it is now doubted that this is so. Although both retinol and its derivatives, the retinoids, are being increasingly used in various dermatoses (acne, psoriasis, etc.), there is little evidence that vitamin A deficiency produces any recognizable skin abnormality.

Vitamin B Deficiencies

Beriberi

Thiamine is particularly necessary for the maintenance of the nervous system and the heart. Deficient intake may produce neuromuscular changes (with or without edema) or cardiovascular conditions. The edematous form, known as wet beriberi, was common in Southeast Asia, particularly in the prisons of Singapore and Malaya, but when polished rice in the diet was changed to the unpolished type the disease rapidly disappeared and is now rare.

Changes in the nervous system may produce wrist-drop or foot-drop, which can be confused with neural leprosy, but the deficiency is unlikely to produce any dermatologic change.

Pellagra

This condition is caused by a deficiency of nicotinic acid and is particularly frequent where maize is the dietary staple. Although it may be associated with other symptoms, it is classically supposed to show the "three-D syndrome"— dementia, dermatitis, and diarrhea.

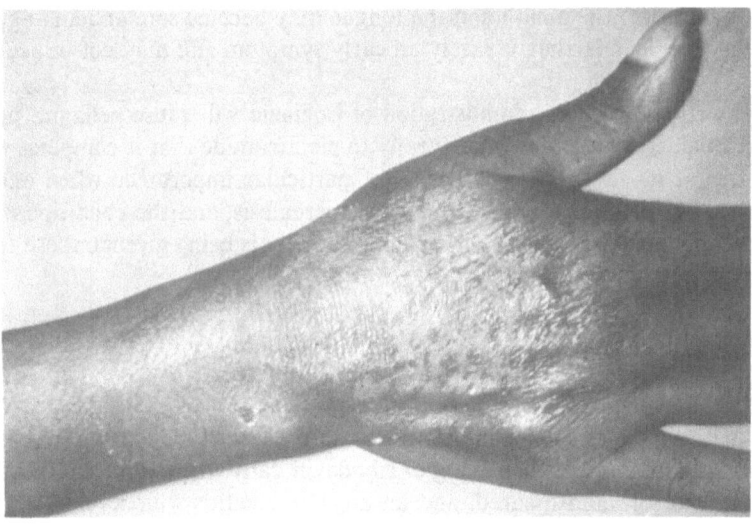

FIGURE 28-2   Pellagra: scaling and hyperpigmentation on hand.

The dementia is usually mild, amounting to little more than depression, but sometimes frankly psychotic behavior is seen, which responds rapidly to intravenous nicotinic acid. The skin eruption, a dramatic mixture of dryness and hyperpigmentation, is usually confined to the sun-exposed areas—the backs of the hands (Figure 28-2) and the face—while classically a well-defined eruption surrounds the front of the neck to give the "pellagra necklace" (Figure 28-3).

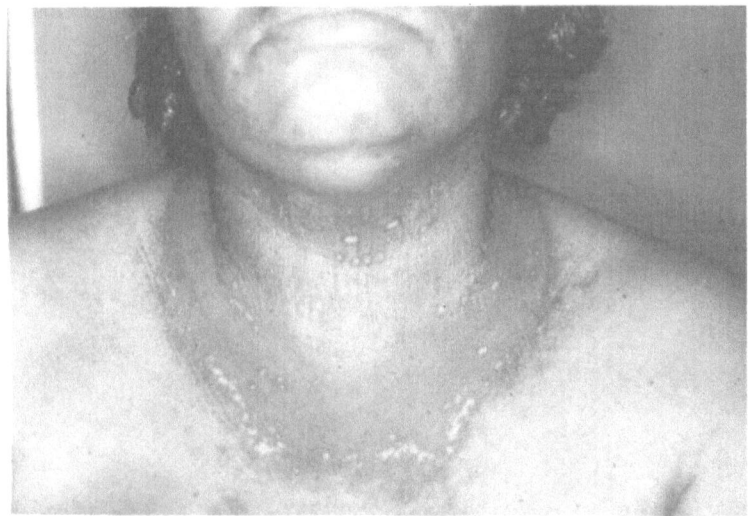

FIGURE 28-3   Pellagra: necklace.

At the same time the mouth and the tongue may become sore and an angular cheilitis develop. Diarrhea is rarely an early symptom and may not be seen at all.

It is well known that administration of isoniazid will cause pellagra, probably because it is so similar structurally to nicotinamide that it competes with the latter at its site of action. This is of particular importance when undernourished patients are being treated for tuberculosis, and the condition must be especially guarded against when such treatment is being given to those Indians who are strict vegetarians.

Ariboflavinosis

The main sources of riboflavin are meat and milk. If the dietary intake is so low that it contains less than 2 mg of riboflavin daily, the tongue will become raw, the lips sore and fissured, and an angular cheilitis will develop. At the same time an acute eczematous eruption may appear on the scrotum.

Treatment

As vitamin B deficiencies often appear in combination rather than individually, it is safer to treat them all with compound vitamin B tablets containing thiamin, riboflavin, and nicotinic acid.

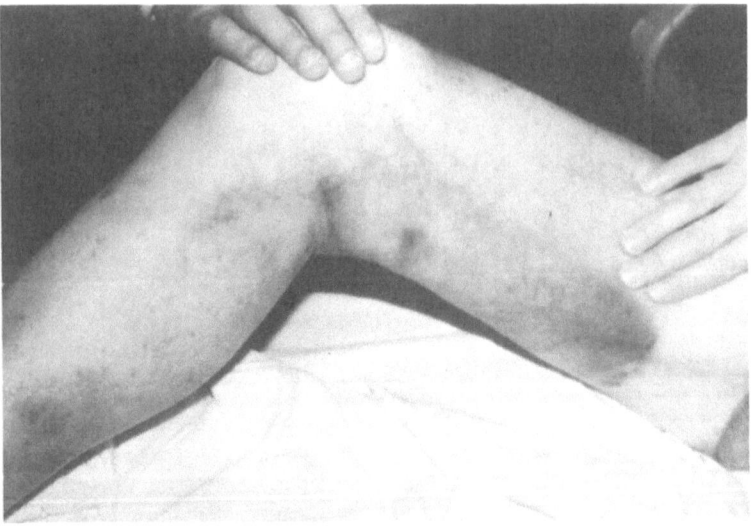

FIGURE 28-4   Scurvy: note ecchymosis and perifollicular hemorrhages, which can be confused with purpura. (Courtesy Dr. Thomas Connolly, Philadelphia, Pennsylvania.)

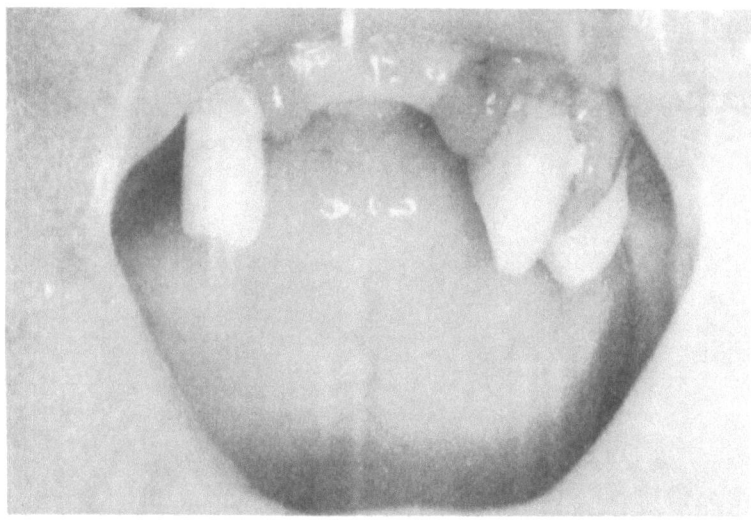

FIGURE 28-5   Scurvy: the characteristic swollen edentulous gums. (Courtesy Dr. Thomas Connolly, Philadelphia, Pennsylvania.)

Vitamin C Deficiency

Lack of vitamin C is not particularly common in tropical zones, but in subtropical areas where fresh fruit and vegetables are scarce, scurvy may be seen. It is probably more frequent in Europe, where it affects those elderly people, living alone, who limit their diet to what is cheap and easy to prepare and destroy their vitamin C supply (if any) by boiling vegetables.

Scurvy starts with a loss of weight. Corkscrew hairs appear on the shins while changes in vascular permeability produce perifollicular hemorrhages that may be confused with purpura (Figure 28-4). Later, larger ecchymoses are seen, and if bleeding affects the joints a painful arthritis soon develops. In the mouth, swollen and perhaps bleeding gums are among the earliest signs (Figure 28-5).

Relatively small doses of vitamin C (100 mg daily) will soon produce clinical improvement, but the ecchymoses will fade only slowly and the joints may be permanently stiffened.

Selected Readings

Brock, JF, Autret, M: Kwashiorkor in Africa. *Bull WHO* 1952; 5:1.

Meyrick-Thomas, RH, Payne, CMER, Black, MM: Isoniazid induced pellagra. *Br Med J* 1981; 283:297.

Sandozia, MK, Haquani, AH, Rajesheri, V, Jasbir,K: Kwashiorkor. *Br Med J* 1963; 2:83.

Wells, GC: Skin diseases in relation to malabsorption. *Br Med J* 1962; 2:937.

Williams, CD: A nutritional disease of childhood associated with a maize diet. *Arch Dis Child* 1933; 8:423.

CHAPTER 29

Phrynoderma

In 1933, Loewenthal, writing from Africa, and Nicholls, in South India, described almost simultaneously a condition they both attributed to vitamin A deficiency. Nicholls suggested the name phrynoderma, meaning toad skin, and defined it as "a papular dry skin eruption, frequently being accompanied by mild neuritis and or eye symptoms. The patients are very liable to diarrhea and dysentery, and when this occurs, the neuritis becomes worse." It was not unknown for this combination of symptoms to prove fatal.

Since that time, the skin condition has been persistently recognized, more commonly in the tropics than elsewhere, but nowadays the systemic ill health that seemed to be an essential accompaniment to the eruption is rarely if ever found.

Etiology

In 1933, the condition was attributed to vitamin A deficiency, as the skin lesions were associated with night blindness and xerophthalmia. When an ounce of cod-liver oil was administered daily to a series of more than 80 patients, all the cases of night blindness got better and all but one of the skin lesions. Some years later, however, it was reported that not everybody improved with vitamin A; some only improved when their protein intake was increased and vitamin B was given. In the 1960s, a discussion arose as to whether the condition was caused by a general vitamin B deficiency or a specific lack of riboflavin. Most patients diagnosed as having phrynoderma today are not suffering from any recognizable deficiency, and the etiology remains a mystery.

Clinical Features

In the tropics, most of the patients are under the age of 16. They have dome-shaped polygonal or circular papules consisting of distended follicles plugged with keratin, which are on average from 1 to 3 mm in diameter (Figure 29-1). The eruption is first seen on the extensor surfaces of the limbs, particularly the knees and elbows, and it slowly spreads to other parts of the limbs but is relatively rare on the trunk or face. Frequently, the papules cluster in more or less circular patches 3 to 5 cm in diameter. These areas often show obviously hypopigmented in comparison with the normal skin. Sometimes, especially if the eruption is unusually extensive, the hypopigmented background is less clearly noticeable (Figure 29-2).

The original descriptions made great play of the associated symptoms, eye changes, dysentery, and marasmus, which frequently lead to death. These other symptoms are not seen today, although the skin lesions seem to be indistinguishable from the original descriptions.

Differential Diagnosis

Phrynoderma is a member of that spectrum of follicular keratoses that ranges from the small, scaly papules often called keratosis pilaris, which spread diffusely over the trunk and limbs, to keratosis spinulosa, which probably only

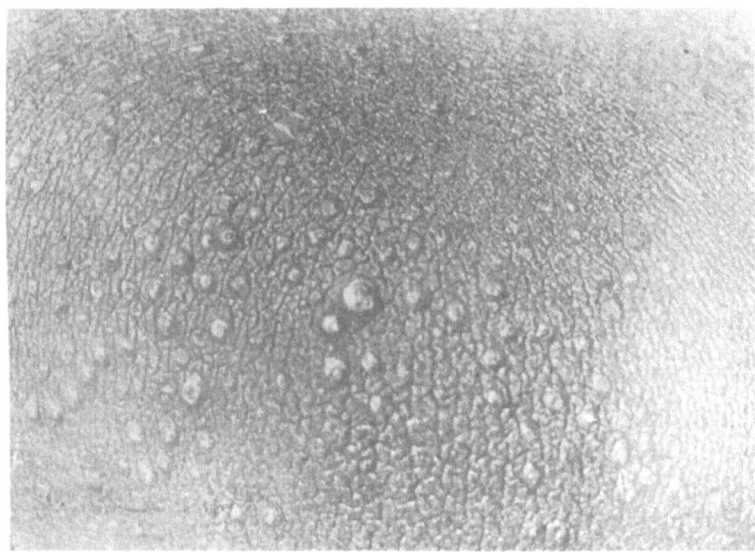

FIGURE 29-1   Dome-shaped, plugged papules characteristic of phrynoderma.

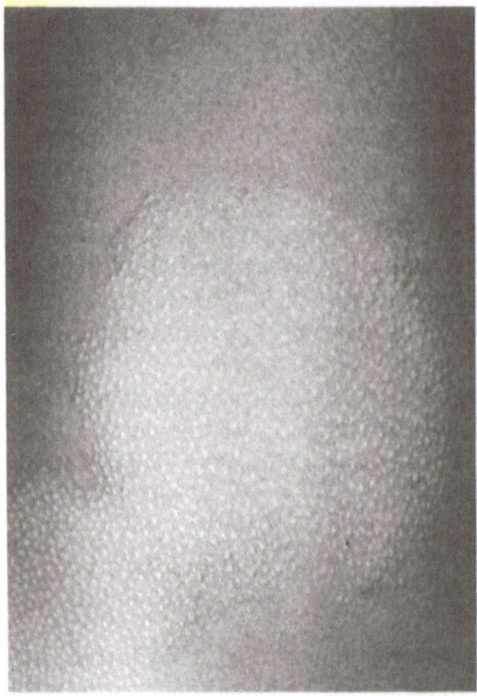

FIGURE 29-2   Grouped follicular keratoses.

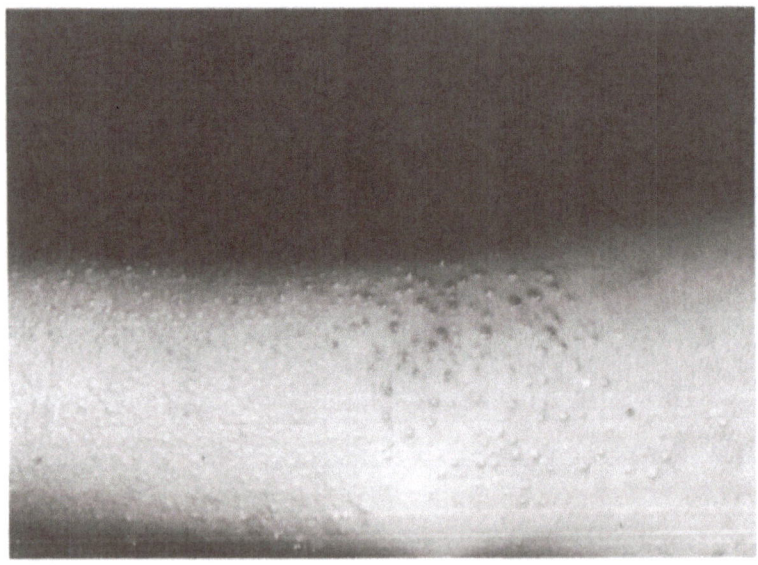

FIGURE 29-3   Follicular lesions that resemble lichen spinulosus.

differs from phrynoderma in that the horny plug protrudes from the follicle in a spiky way. Sometimes, both the dome-shaped lesions of phrynoderma and the pointed ones of lichen spinulosus may be seen alongside each other on the same part of the skin (Figure 29-3).

Pityriasis rubra pilaris has a somewhat similar histologic appearance but is associated with sufficiently dramatic clinical signs elsewhere for the diagnosis not to be confused, while lichen planopilaris, if it occurs in the absence of the diagnostic cicatricial alopecia, may cause problems of diagnosis that can only be clarified by histologic examination.

The histology shows just what might be clinically expected: a laminated, horny plug distending the upper part of a follicle.

Treatment

At various times the use of vitamins has apparently been extremely effective for this condition, but today it seems to respond poorly, if at all, to such therapy. It may even be suspected that, despite the clinical similarities, the toad-skin eruption seen now has a different etiology than that which was seen in association with the general state of malnutrition that occurred in Africa and India during the colonial era.

Mild cases respond slowly to the local application of 2 to 3 percent salicylic acid and 2 to 3 percent sulfur in a zinc cream base, while larger lesions, more comedonal in appearance, often improve with the use of 0.05 percent retinoic acid (tretinoin). This may be too irritating for younger patients, and it can be diluted with an equal amount of hydrocortisone cream or another of the weaker corticosteroids.

The condition is rarely seen in patients over 20 years of age, and it is suspected that many cases improve without medical assistance.

Selected Readings

Loewenthal, LJA: A new cutaneous manifestation in the syndrome of vitamin A deficiency. *Arch Dermatol Syphilol* 1933; 28:700.

Nicholls, L: Phrynoderma: A condition due to vitamin deficiency. *Indian Med Gaz* 1933; 68:681.

Pettit, JHS: Phrynoderma. *Int J Dermatol* 1983; 22:117.

Shrank, AB: Phrynoderma. *Br Med J* 1966; 1:29.

Chapter 30

Brazilian Pemphigus Foliaceous

The words *pemphigus braziliensis* were used two centuries ago to describe a bullous disease that was found primarily in Brazil and that has now been recognized in the adjoining countries of Bolivia, Peru, Venezuela, and Uruguay. Sometimes known as fogo selvagem (wild fire) and even confused with Tokelau ringworm (*T. concentricum*), it is now realized that in many ways the condition is indistinguishable from pemphigus foliaceous. There are, however, enough dissimilarities to suggest that Brazilian pemphigus foliaceous may be a distinct entity. The very high incidence (over 700 cases seen in Brazil in 1974 alone), the frequent appearance in the young (one-third of all cases start the disease before they are 20 years old), and the numerous cases with a family history are all features that suggest the diseases are not quite the same.

Most patients come from the rural areas of Brazil. The state of São Paulo had so many patients that a special hospital was built in the main city, but with the urbanization of the area, the incidence diminished and now the state of Goiás has the most cases. There is no difference in sex or race of patients, but there is a predominance of the disease in those people living in agricultural areas.

Etiology

Like pemphigus foliaceous, the cause of Brazilian pemphigus foliaceous is unknown. There have been a number of proponents of the theory that there is a viral etiology. Koch's postulates were in part confirmed when Beutner et al. produced acantholytic bullae in monkeys that had been inoculated with serum from Brazilian cases. As is not unusual with diseases that show a distinct regional localization, insect bites have also been blamed; many patients report having been previously bitten with borrachudos, a member of the Simuliidae, well known in Brazil.

Clinical Features

When the disease is fully established, it is characterized by an extensive symmetric, scaly eruption (Figure 30-1) amounting almost to an erythroderma (Figure 30-2). Scattered throughout these patches but perhaps rather more often found at the periphery are flaccid bullae whose superficial situation in the epidermis is demonstrated by their brief existence—the roof is rapidly rubbed off but the scaling and the erythema remain (Figure 30-3).

New bullae continue to erupt and scaliness is widespread, frequently affecting the whole of the scalp and matting the hair, giving a clinical picture similar to, but more extensive than, tinea amiantacea, which may be followed by a widespread diffuse alopecia. Large patches of erythema on the butterfly area of the face may be complicated by hyperpigmentation, while papillomatosis may be seen on the flexures (axillae, groins, or even the retroauricular folds). Later, palmar-plantar hyperkeratoses are frequently found.

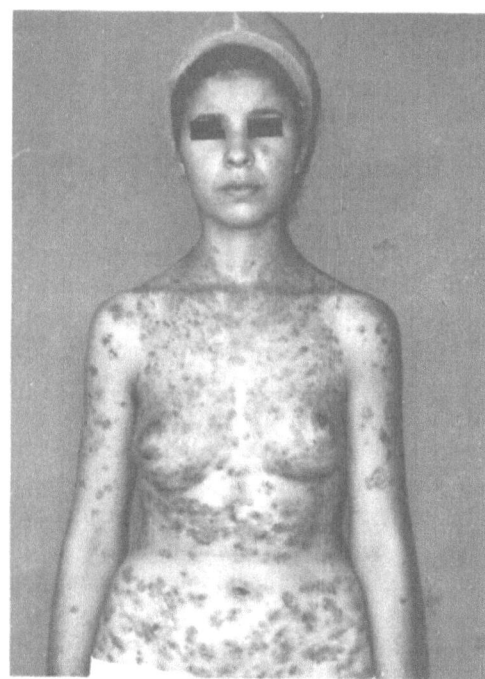

FIGURE 30-1   Symmetrical scaling lesions. (Courtesy Sebastião Sampaio M.D., São Paulo, Brazil.)

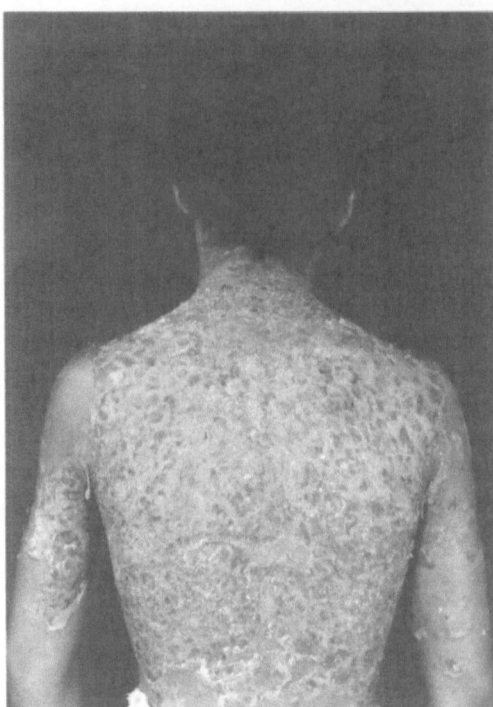

FIGURE 30-2 Diffuse scaling resembling erythroderma. (Courtesy Sebastião Sampaio, M.D., São Paulo, Brazil.

Natural History

The earliest lesions often look more like the Senear-Usher syndrome than a true case of pemphigus foliaceous, starting as it does with a scaly erythema on the face, scalp, and the presternal skin on which few if any vesicles are visible; even at this time, Nikolsky's sign (see Appendix one) is positive. This localized form may persist unchanged for months or years. Sometimes, it has been known to resolve spontaneously, the patient having no further trouble.

More often, the eruption extends insidiously, and slowly the classic picture evolves with erythema, scaling, and bullae anywhere or everywhere on the skin. At the same time the dermatologic lesions may be accompanied by general malaise, nocturnal fever, diarrhea, and amenorrhea. Sometimes, secondary infection of the skin is followed by septicemia and infection in internal organs. In the extensive presence of such immunocompromised skin, it is not surprising that viral contamination has been known to cause Kaposi's varicelliform eruption, while scabies, fungal infections, and warts may all complicate the clinical appearance.

Ultimately, the skin is extensively thickened and hyperpigmented, the nails become discolored and deformed, the sexual organs atrophy, muscles become

FIGURE 30-3 Typical scaling and crusitn in a seven-year-old Brazilian boy. (Courtesy Sebastião Sampaio, M.D., São Paulo, Brazil.)

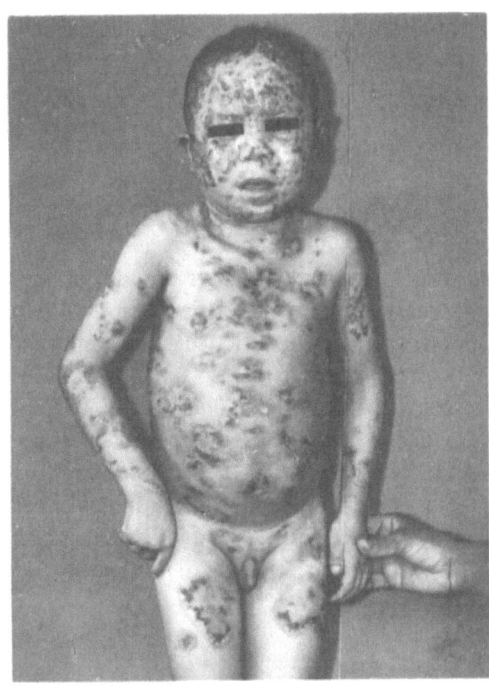

weakened, numerous endocrinopathies appear, and if untreated, death follows in at least 50 percent of the cases.

Differential Diagnosis

Many authors believe that this is simply a variant of pemphigus foliaceous. Both begin on the face and can initially mimic the Senear-Usher syndrome, and they continue to be clinically and histologically undifferentiable from each other. Nowhere else in the world is there an endemic form of pemphigus. Only the Brazilian disease has a high percentage of natural remissions. These distinctions are academic, and all patients should be treated. There is so far little evidence that these diseases, different or not, respond differently to routine therapy.

Other forms of pemphigus (pemphigus vulgaris, pemphigus vegetans, etc.) usually have a more rapid course, with large, tense bullae rather than the small flaccid ones of pemphigus erythematosus—histologically the bulla is sited closer to the basal layer.

The polymorphic dermatitis herpetiformis, with its symmetrical distribution, could perhaps be confused clinically, but it is rare in Brazil, and the histology and immunology are totally different.

Investigations

The diagnosis can be established by histologic examination of a bulla. In all cases of pemphigus, acantholysis occurs in the epidermis but here the acantholytic split is in the upper part in, or just below, the granular layer. If for any reason the patient refuses a biopsy, a Tzanck test (see appendix one) will demonstrate acantholytic cells on the floor of the bulla.

If facilities are available for immunofluorescent studies, direct immunofluorescence will reveal positive pemphigus antibodies. IgG is common and C_3 not infrequent. Indirect immunofluorescence is usually positive in established cases but may be negative in the earlier, Senear-Usher-like phase.

It is interesting to note that antiepithelial antibodies have been detected in healthy people living in endemic areas. This lends credence to the possibility that the disease is etiologically different from ordinary pemphigus foliaceous.

Treatment

As spontaneous recovery cannot be relied upon, all diagnosed cases must be treated. It is usually recommended that oral corticosteroids be used, starting with fairly high doses equivalent to 100 mg of prednisone a day until all new lesions have been suppressed. The dosage may be slowly reduced until more bullae start to appear, at which time a mildly raised dosage must be sustained for a few weeks until diminishing therapy can be reintroduced. Within six months, it is usually possible to maintain the patient on one or two tablets a day.

As with all other patients needing prolonged high doses of corticosteroids, it seems to be wiser to give the drug as a single dose on alternate days. Such treatment is believed to reduce the side effects of the drug, which may, in long-term medication, be as dangerous as the disease itself.

An alternative therapy is to give quinacrine 0.3 to 0.6 g daily for several months, but chloroquine is not so useful.

It should also be remembered that patients are not necessarily exempt from other diseases. In Brazil more than 10 percent of the patients have associated pulmonary tuberculosis. It is, of course, imperative that this should be energetically treated. If possible, corticosteroids should be withheld and quinacrine used until the tuberculosis has been inactivated. In such circumstances, it may be helpful to supplement therapy with the special tar paint that was used before the introduction of corticosteroids. It is called jamarsan R and consists of the following ingredients:

Sulfur ppt	150 g
Zinc oxide powder	120 g
Boric acid powder	100 g
Calcium hydroxide	100 g
Turpentine	15 g
Crude coal tar	3,000 g
Cottonseed oil	1,500 g

It may be applied twice weekly all over the body for several months.

Selected Readings

Azulay, RD: Brazilian pemphigus foliaceous. *Int J Dermatol* 1982; 21:122.

Beutner, EH, Prigenzi, LS, Hale, W, et al: Immunofluorescent studies of auto-antibodies to intercellular areas of epithelia in Brazilian pemphigus foliaceous. *Proc Soc Exp Biol Med* 1968; 127:81.

Beutner, EH, Wood, GW, Chorzelski, GP, et al: Produção de lesões semelhantes às do Pênfigo foliáceo pela injeção intradérmica am coelhos e macacos, de soros de doentes com titulo elevado de autoanticorpe. *Mem Inst Butantan* 1971; 35:79.

Brown, MV: Fogo selvagem (Pemphigus foliaceus): Review of the Brazilian literature. *AMA Arch Dermatol Syphilol* 1954; 69:589.

Castro, RM, Roscoe, JT, Sampaio, SAP: Brazilian Pemphigus foliaceus. *Clin Dermatol* 1983; 1(2):22.

Martins-Castro, R, Proenca, N, de Salles-Gomes, LF: On the association of some dermatoses with South American pemphigus foliaceus. *Int J Dermatol* 1974; 13:271.

Sevadjian, C: Nosology of brazilian pemphigus foliaceus. *Int J Dermatol* 1979; 17:781.

CHAPTER 31

Chronic Arsenical Poisoning

There are three ways in which people may swallow arsenic in sufficient doses to produce signs of chronic poisoning. First, there may be some criminal interference in the diet, although the wish to exterminate one's enemies with arsenic seems to arise less frequently than it did 100 years ago. In any case, it would be a bungling murderer who gave low doses for such a long time that the vicim developed chronic arsenism. Second, and also increasingly unusual, medical practitioners may supply arsenic to their patients as a tonic or as treatment for psoriasis, lichen planus, or syphilis. Fowler's solution is not a modern form of therapy, but patients may still be found who were given long courses of therapeutic arsenic 30, 40, or 50 years ago. Quacks have also used arsenic as a panacea. In Ireland they sold it as a cure for cancer. Finally, there are sporadic reports of chronic arsenical intoxication following the use of contaminated drinking water, occurring in groups with a few individuals to a few hundred. These cases are almost invariably focused around contaminated wells.

In northern Iran dozens of people were affected when a leaking drain from the public bath affected a series of nearby wells. In the bath, the villagers had used a locally applied arsenical paste as a pubic hair depilatory. Foci are known to have occurred in Malaysia in wells that have been sunk in the neighborhood of tin mines (when tin is removed from the ground, other elements remain in increased percentages).

Contamination of natural water supply was recognized as early as 1913 in Argentina and has been reported more recently from Taiwan and from Oregon in the United States.

Etiology

Although most outbreaks occur in sites where the arsenical content of the available water is higher than it should be, occasional patients seem to develop chronic arsenism, when the arsenic in their water supply is within permitted limits. It is obvious that no one can be poisoned who has no contact with the chemical, but it may be that there is an individual metabolic trait that plays a part in the retention of arsenic in tissue. A number of patients with arsenically induced carcinomata were given arsenic by mouth. The urinary excretion was lower in carcinoma subjects than in others, suggesting a tendency to increased storage. This work has not been repeated.

As early as 1888, Hutchison reported six cases of malignancy in patients whose neoplastic changes were attributed to the therapeutic ingestion of potassium arsenite. In 1922 Leach showed that metastasizing tumors followed repeated application of potassium arsenite to rat skin. It is possible that these malignancies were particularly associated with the use of inorganic arsenical preparations. It is not clear whether the organic trivalent and pentavalent arsenicals are also to blame. Probably, the arsenic in such formulations is stable, being attached to a benzene ring, which does not usually liberate organic arsenic into the system.

Clinical Features

The lesions on the skin usually appear after several years of low-grade arsenical ingestion; because of this, the condition is rare in children. At first, a slowly increasing hyperpigmentation appears, affecting large areas of the skin, particularly on the front or back of the trunk. The scapular areas and limbs are involved later. This slate-grey pigmentation is usually fairly uniform, but less frequently it can be patchy. Often, small guttate areas of normal skin are scattered through the diffuse melanosis. They are compared to raindrops on a dusty road and are sometimes mistakenly taken for hypopigmented areas on a normal skin; a careful search for the edge of the discoloration will reveal normal skin for comparison.

Arsenical keratoses develop in every poisoned patient, even if there is little or no evidence of preceding melanoderms. Scattered lesions on the soles (Figure 31-1), palms (Figure 31-2), or fingers may look like warts but are usually

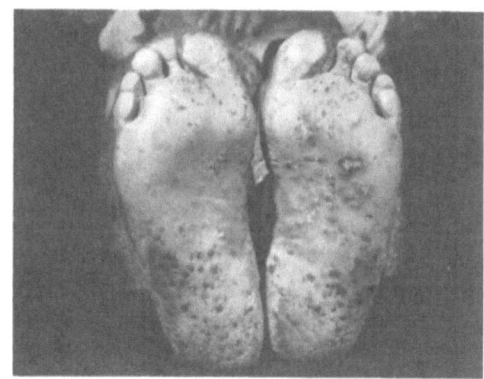

FIGURE 31-1 Keratotic lesions dotting the soles. (Courtesy Stephanie Jablonska, M.D., Warsaw, Poland.)

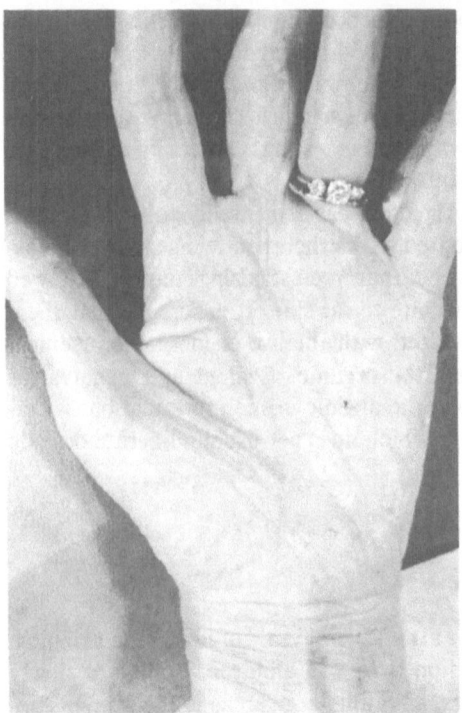

FIGURE 31-2   Keratosis and scaling on the palms. (Courtesy Jerome S. Maliner, M.D., Eugene, Oregon.)

more protruberant, although punctate lesions are sometimes found. They are present in such great numbers that confusion with verrucae plantaris is unlikely. A surprising number of patients have palmar or plantar hyperidrosis, a finding that has not been explained, but when occurring with multiple keratoses is strongly indicative of arsenism.

As time goes on, carcinomas of the skin will develop. They do not usually start in association with the keratoses, but can be found anywhere on the body. Bowen's disease, oral leukoplakia, basal cell carcinoma, squamous cell carcinoma, and keratoacanthoma may all be seen alone or in any combination all over the skin.

Differential Diagnosis

There is not much problem in reaching a clinical diagnosis of chronic arsenism, if the history is available; unless arsenic has been administered therapeutically, almost all the patients will say that other members of their family are involved. In Iran the community believed the palmar-plantar keratoses to be infectious, because "if somebody gets it, all his family gets it too." It is also useful to know whether a patient comes from an area where other cases of arsenism have been recognized.

The keratoses have to be differentiated from other forms of plantar keratosis, which usually appear earlier in life, while Darier's disease affects the trunk as well as the palms. Tylosis palmaris et plantaris is more diffuse, acrokeratosis verruciformis is more marked on the dorsum of the hands, and epidermodysplasia verruciformis is a generalized disease where there are flat and elevated warty lesions in many sites.

The slate-grey pigmentation, which in some patients has a more golden tinge, might be confused with a whole range of hereditary and acquired hypermelanoses. Although the raindrop appearance is suggestive of arsenism, other dyschromatoses may also show a mottled look. The presence of arsenical keratoses clinches the diagnosis.

Investigations

If the suspicion of arsenism has been aroused, analysis of the urine will show arsenic to be present if the ingestion is continuing, and proof of arsenic remains in the hair and nails for 2 to 3 years after ingestion has stopped.

The histology, if such facilities are available, will show the types of abnormalities that are expected (dyskeratoses, dysplasias, and epitheliomata) but little or no evidence of their arsenical origin, although Lever suggests that vacuolization of epidermal cells (two or three times as large as normal) may be seen in arsenical keratoses. If such cells occur in considerable numbers in squamous cell carcinoma, the lesion is of arsenical origin.

Treatment

Once started, none of the serious manifestations ever regresses, although there may in time be a fading of the melanoderma. The gravest complications are the external and internal malignancies. Clinical attention must be principally directed to them.

Arsenical keratoses do not respond to topical 5-fluorouracil, and they are best handled by the local use of 20 percent salicylic acid. Ten percent urea cream sometimes helps, and we know of patients who smooth down their soles with sandpaper.

Prophylaxis should be easy in any country, where the public health authorities take their work seriously. As soon as a focus of contamination has been recognized the sources of water must be examined and any that are affected should be permanently sealed. In the United States, more than 0.05 mg per liter is considered unsafe, and in Britain the arsenical content of water is not allowed to excede 0.1 mg per liter. A reliable piped water supply must be provided for the area and the inhabitants must be continually reminded that contaminated water is not improved by boiling.

Follow-up

Patients whose poisoning ceased many years before will still show melanoderma, keratoses, and malignancies. There is little evidence that cessation of intoxication reverses the inexorable process of arsenism. The importance of the condition does not only lie in the fact that chronic arsenism leads to a range of dermatologic abnormalities.

A 1978 study of a group of patients who had been treated with arsenic in the 1930s showed a significant increase in the incidence of malignant internal neoplasms, mainly in the lungs and gastrointestinal tract. As this finding has been known for many years in Argentina and is the subject of sporadic reports from other countries, it is essential that all cases of chronic arsenism be followed indefinitely.

Patients must be warned that regular checkups are imperative if possible complications are to be detected at an early stage.

Selected Readings

Bettley, FR, O'Shea, JD: The absorption of arsenic and its relation to carcinoma. *Br J Dermatol* 1975; 92:563.

Reymann, F, Moller, R, Nielsen, A: Relationship between arsenical intake and internal malignancy. *Arch Dermatol* 1978; 114:378.

Tseng, WP, Chu, HM, How, Sw, et al: Prevalence of skin cancer in an endemic area of chronic arsenicism in Taiwan. *J Natl Cancer Inst* 1968; 40:453.

Wagner, SL, Maliner, JS, Morton, WE, et al: Skin cancer and arsenical intoxication from well-water. *Arch Dermatol* 1979; 115:1205.

Useful Techniques

In the body of this book, many investigations have been recommended that are of help in confirming the various diagnoses. Many of these (routine histology, bacteriology) are well known to most readers, but we suspect that others are less widely used. This appendix contains details of a number of procedures that may be helpful to the nonspecialist.

Cellophane Tape Test

Transparent self-adhesive plastic tape (Cellotape, Scotch tape) is extremely useful in confirming the diagnosis of pityriasis versicolor. Three to four centimeters of the tape are stuck over an active area and firmly rubbed with the back of a fingernail. When removed, the tape will show an exact replica of the scaly lesion that it has covered. This in itself is diagnostic of pityriasis versicolor, but further confirmation can be obtained if the tape is dipped for one minute into a drop of 1 percent gentian violet, blotted, and mounted on a microscope slide. Examination will show the spores and germ tubes of the *Pityrosporum*.

The cellophane tape test is negative in early cases of tinea imbricata, which may sometimes be confused with pityriasis versicolor.

Diascopy

It is often helpful to know whether or not a dermal papule has a vascular element. This can best be recognized by determining whether it blanches on pressure, but as the pressing finger will entirely cover a small lesion, it is more helpful if the pressure is exerted with some hard, flat material that is transparent. This permits the nodule to be seen while it is under pressure. Such instruments may be a plastic tongue depressor or spatula, a magnifying lens, or some other reasonably thick piece of glass. An ordinary microscope slide can be used, but they have been known to break under pressure and lacerate the patient.

Diascopy is of particular value in examination of nodules in a patient suspected of having lupus vulgaris. The apple-jelly nodule is often rather erythematous, and only under diascopy will the typical greenish-yellow color be clearly revealed.

The Matchstick Test

An even older technique for demonstrating an apple-jelly nodule, located in the upper part of the dermis, and covered by a taut, stretched epidermis, involves taking an ordinary wooden match that has been sharpened to a point and placing it vertical to the papule. Light pressure with a finger will cause the match to penetrate the epidermis and stand upright without support. If the lesion is deep in the dermis and the epidermis is not thinned, the point of the match will break under pressure.

Both these tests are positive in lupus vulgaris and lupoid leishmaniasis and negative in tuberculoid granulomata.

Dutz Technique

For the many bacterial or parasitic lesions that show crusting or ulceration, cotton swabs are usually used to obtain suitable material for examination or culture. This method is often ineffective in ulcerated lesions and of no use at all if a sample is needed from the depths of a dermal infection. It is better to use a dental broach. These instruments, used by dentists to abrade dentine, are steel needles, the distal part being surrounded by metallic barbs of different sizes. The finer broaches may easily be pushed into the core of an infected area, producing a very small puncture wound. If they are gently rotated before removal, they will become coated with tissue, which can be used for a stab culture, to make a direct smear for bacteriologic examination, or to inoculate a bacterial plate.

If the lesion is crusted, it is usually possible to insert the broach from the side into the main body of the swelling and so completely avoid any surface contamination that may be present. The technique has been found useful for leishmaniasis, leprosy, anthrax, and yaws. (Reference: Dutz, W, Kohout, E: Dermatologic diagnosis by using the hemocytometer and the dental broach. *Int J Dermatol* 1982; 21:410.)

Lepromin Test

If lepromin is available and kept at a suitable temperature, it can be used as a diagnostic aid. It seems to have become traditional to use the left forearm some two inches distal to the elbow fold to inject 0.1 ml intradermally.

Although the WHO suggests that readings should be taken after 28 days, those taken after three weeks are acceptable. The diameter of the resultant papule is measured in millimeters and recorded.

0–3 mm	negative
3–6 mm	+
6–9 mm	+ +
Over 10 mm	+ + +

Unfortunately, both false negative and false positive reactions are possible, the former perhaps because the injection has been too deep and the latter because an unclean needle has caused a small intradermal infection.

The combination of clinical, bacteriologic, and histopathologic findings usually makes the lepromin an unnecessary luxury.

Leprosy Skin Smear

It may be impossible to detect any *M. leprae* in a lesion of tuberculoid leprosy, but in all other types the mycobacterium is present in varying numbers. The demonstration of its presence is an essential part of the clinical investigation of borderline and lepromatous disease.

How to Do the Skin-Slit

The following equipment is necessary:

1. a supply of clean, preferably unused microscope slides;
2. an alcohol lamp;
3. numerous gauze or cotton swabs;
4. 1 percent cetrimide or other nonflammable skin cleanser;
5. a scalpel handle fitted with a No. 15 Bard Parker blade.

The purpose of this investigation is to detect the presence of leprosy organisms. It is not a blood test. The lesion should be squeezed between the forefinger and thumb of one hand until it is suitably blanched. The skin is then cleaned, an incision 3 to 4 mm long is made, and, the blade being turned at right angles, one of the walls of the cut is firmly scraped to remove a drop of tissue fluid. This is smeared onto a clean slide over an area approximately 1 cm in diameter (two or three smears can be made on each slide). If the lesion has been firmly held, the smear will not be bloodstained. Sometimes the incision will bleed after the smear has been taken—a small wisp of cotton will ensure rapid coagulation.

The scalpel blade is wiped with cetrimide, flamed on the alcohol lamp, and cleaned again before the next smear is taken. Which sites are studied should be recorded so that further investigations in three or six months' time will be from the same lesions and so be truly comparable.

Where to Do the Skin-Slit

Patients in the borderline group (BT, BB, or BL) will not have a generalized eruption, and there is no point in taking smears from skin that is not clinically and visibly involved. Six different sites should be tested to obtain an overall picture of the activity and severity of the disease. For lepromatous patients, the following routine is recommended. The shirtless patient sits on a stool with his back to the operator and smears are taken from the following sites:

1. left ear lobe;
2. right ear lobe;
3. lesion from the back of the left arm;
4. lesion somewhere on the back;
5. lesion from the right arm;
6. the patient turning toward the operator, lesion on the knee or thigh.

It is helpful to take smears from both ear lobes, because the unexpected presence of bacilli can be taken as evidence that the patient's disease is becoming completely lepromatous.

This technique is not particularly scientific, as an unmeasured quantity of fluid is smeared over an unmeasured area on the slide; different operators will produce smears that differ widely in thickness. It is urged that a patient's smears always be taken by the same operator, thus minimizing the possibility of extensive technical variation.

How to Count the Skin-Slit

All smears should be fixed by gentle heating and then stained. Four solutions are needed:

Solution A   10 percent carbol fuchsin in 90 percent absolute alcohol
Solution B   5 percent phenol in 95 percent distilled water
Solution C   0.5 percent hydrochloric acid in 70 percent alcohol
Solution D   1 percent methylene blue

Step 1

Combine 1 ml of solution A with 9 ml of solution B and cover the smear for 20 minutes. It may be gently heated, but not dried out, for a minute at the start of staining. After this, the slide should be washed with running water.

Step 2

Decolorize the smear by pouring on a small amount of solution C for a few seconds and wash again with running water. If the smear is still red, decolorize further, until there is nothing left but a pale pink tinge.

Step 3

Counterstain with solution D for two minutes, wash and leave to dry.

The stain is now ready to be counted. Under an oil-immersion lens, the mycobacteria should appear as red-stained rods. Other tissues are slightly blue. Ridley's logarithmic index is used to count the organisms. One hundred oil-immersion fields are examined on each smear, and the total number of bacilli are recorded as follows:

1–9 organisms in 100 fields	1+
10–99 organisms in 100 fields	2+
1–9 organisms in every field	3+
10–99 organisms in every field	4+
More than 100 organisms in every field	5+

It is possible but very unusual to find more than 1,000 bacilli in each field. This must be counted as 6+.

The bacterial index (BI) is then recorded as the average from all the six sites examined.

What to Count

Unfortunately, even with successful antileprosy treatment the BI takes a very long time to diminish significantly, as dead *M. leprae* are astonishingly slow to disintegrate. Three or six monthly estimations of the BI do not give a satisfactory record of the patient's progress. Fortunately, under the oil-immersion lens it can be seen that all bacteria do not take the stain in the same way—some bacilli show uniform coloration while others appear fragmented and granular. It is now known that only the uniform staining bacteria are viable. Use of this knowledge is another method of measurement, called the morphologic index (MI). In most untreated cases, 20 to 30 percent of all the bacilli stain uniformly. A few weeks after the onset of therapy this percentage will fall to zero. Reduction in the MI precedes by several months a fall in the BI. Thus, the MI will show whether or not treatment is being successful.

While the BI is being counted the MI should be estimated at the same time.

One hundred consecutive separately visible organisms should be examined and the percentage of those that are solidly staining recorded. If six smears are taken, the average of the bacterial and the morphologic indices will give a general statement of the patient's condition. If after several months of supposedly efficacious therapy the MI has not decreased, either the patient is not taking the treatment or there is a drug-resistant organism (Reference: Leiker, DL, McDougall, AC: Technical guide for smear examination for leprosy by direct microscopy. Amsterdam Leprosy Documentation Service, 1983.)

Nikolsky's Sign

This sometimes helps to differentiate pemphigus from other bullous diseases. The sign, described by Nikolsky in 1895, is elicited by exerting firm sliding pressure with a finger on a patient's apparently normal skin. The sign is positive if there is resulting dislodgement of some or all of the epidermis in the pressure area. Gentle, direct pressure on a vesicle or a bulla may cause lateral extension of the lesion, but this is not Nikolsky's sign.

In some other conditions, particularly Lyell's toxic epidermal necrolysis, the Nikolsky's sign is also positive, but such cases do not show the acantholytic cells that can be demonstrated by the Tzanck test (see page 249).

Onchocerciasis Skin Snip

The positive detection of microfilariae in the skin is very helpful in the examination of patients thought to have onchocerciasis. A sharp needle is inserted into the epidermis and a "tent" of skin is raised that is then shaved off; efficient practitioners do not cause any bleeding. The snipped piece of epidermis is placed on a drop of saline on a slide and teased out. Microscopic examination will show the presence of the microfilariae.

Test of Viabiity of Schistsoma Ova

Urine

The urine should be centrifuged, and the supernatant rejected. Clean water is added to the sediment and the process repeated as often as necessary until the supernatant fluid is completely clear. The sediment should be kept in a refrigerator overnight, and the next morning warm water added to the tube. The eggs will soon hatch. The highly motile myracidia can be seen easily with a hand lens, particularly if the tube is viewed against a dark background.

Useful Addresses

Culture Media and Laboratory Equipment

General:

Arthur H. Thomas Company
Vine at Third Street
Philadelphia, PA 19106
(01) (215) 574-4500

Dermatologic Lab and Supply Company
201 Ridge
Council Bluffs, IA 51501
(01) (800) 831-6273

Specific:

Baker's DTM
Key Pharmaceuticals, Inc.
P.O. Box 694307
Miami, FL 33169
(01) (800) 327-0592

Surgical Supplies

General:

George Tiemann and Company
80 Newton Plaza
Plainview, NY 11803
(01) (516) 694-6283

Stool

A few grams of feces are emulsified with saline, strained to remove the coarser particles, and allowed to stand. The supernatant fluid is decanted, and the sediment washed repeatedly as described above. Addition of warm water after the sediment has been in a refrigerator will cause the eggs to hatch if they are viable.

NB. Do not forget (especially in endemic areas) that the demonstration of viable ova is no proof that the patient's symptoms are due to schistosomiasis.

Tzanck Test

The classical forms of pemphigus are all caused by acantholysis, in which the cells of the malphighian layer become separated from each other, round off, and are seen lying separately or in groups in the blister fluid. These are easily seen in a histologic section, but some patients are unwilling to submit to biopsy. The Tzanck smear provides a fairly satisfactory alternative method for demonstrating the acantholytic cells.

The roof of an intact bulla is carefully removed, and the floor of the blister is lightly scraped with a sterile (but preferably blunt) scalpel. The tissue is spread onto a slide, fixed, and stained with hematoxylin and eosin. Smears from an active case of pemphigus will contain the diagnostic acantholytic cells. This test is particularly useful in cases of Brazilian pemphigus foliaceous, as workers in rural districts may have a microscope but no access to a histopathology laboratory.

Wood's Light

Certain fungi fluoresce under Wood's light, which is an ultraviolet light, filtered through a nickel-cobalt glass filter. Many forms are available. The easiest one to use resembles a large electric bulb made of blue glass. It can be effective only in a completely dark room and should be turned on for a few minutes to warm up before it is used. Tineas on the body rarely fluoresce, but many of the causative organisms of tinea capitis will do so.

This is of particular value in cases of favus. Adult patients with a patchy cicatricial alopecia may or may not still have an active infection, since the condition does not resolve spontaneously at puberty as happens in other forms of tinea capitis. Under the light, affected hairs show a grey-green fluorescence, and even if only one or two hairs are affected, they can be recognized and submitted to direct microscopy. Without the Wood's light, hairs can only be randomly selected for microscopy, and negative examination will never fully persuade the doctor or the patient that the whole scalp is free from infection. (Reference: Ronchese, F: The Wood light in dermatology. *Cutis* 1968; 4:1059.)

Drugs, Biologicals, and Medical Sundries

General:

Doctors Pharmacy
1935 Chestnut Street
Philadelphia, PA 19103
(01) (215) 563-1930

Mérieux Institute
17 Rue Bourgelay
69002 Lyon, France

Specific:

Anti-parasitic Drugs

Parasitic Disease Drug Service
Center for Disease Control
Atlanta, GA 30333
(01) (404) 329-3311

Medicated Bandages, Elastoplast

T.J. Smith and Nephew Ltd.
Bessemer Road
Welwyn Garden City
Herts AL7 1HF, England

Praziquantel

Miles Pharmaceuticals
400 Morgan Lane
West Haven, CT 06516
(01) (203) 934-9221

Thalidomide (essential for treatment of erythema nodosum leprosum)
Grunenthal GMBH
5190 Stolberg-im-Rheinland, West Germany

Vaccines (Anthrax)

Department of Health and Social Security
Room H211
14 Russell Square
London WC1B 5EP, England

Department of Public Health
State of Michigan
3500 North Logan
P.O. Box 30030
Lansing, MI 48909

Skin-Testing Material

General:

Hollister Stier Laboratories
P.O. Box 3145
Spokane, WA 99220
(01) (800) 992-1120

Society of Interest to Readers

International Society of Tropical Dermatology
Sigfrid A. Muller, M.D., Secretary General
Division of Dermatology
Mayo Clinic
200 First Street, SW
Rochester, MN 55901
(01)(507) 284-3736

Periodicals of Interest to Readers

International Journal of Dermatology
a. by membership in International Society of Tropical Dermatology
b. or by subscription
   J.B. Lippincott Company
   East Washington Square
   Philadelphia, PA 19105
   (01) (800) 638-3030

International Journal of Leprosy
Business and Circulation Office
1262 Broad Street
Bloomfield, NJ 07003

Quarterly Bibliography of Major Tropical Diseases
National Library of Medicine
Bethesda, MD 20014

Index

Abdominal actinomycosis, 126, *see also* Actinomycosis
Actinomyces bovis, 124
Actinomyces israelii, 116, 124–125, 128
Actinomycosis
  clinical features of, 125–126
  diagnosis of, 127
  etiology of, 124–125
  investigations of, 127
  natural history of, 126–127
  treatment and follow-up of, 128
Aflatoxin, 222
Allescheria boydii, 116
Alopecia, 103
  cicatrical, 161
  leprosy, 75
  scarring, 101
Amastigote, 159
Amebiasis
  clinical features of, 179
  diagnosis of, 179–180
  etiology of, 178–179
  investigations of, 181
  natural history of, 179
  treatment and follow-up of, 181–182
Amphotericin B
  for chromomycosis, 111
  for mucocutaneous leishmaniasis, 173
  for North American blastomycosis, 144
  for sportrichosis, 123
Anergic leishmaniasis
  clinical features of, 167
  diagnosis of, 169

investigations of, 170
  natural history of, 167, 169
  treatment of, 170
Anesthesia, of lesions, 52, 53, 63
Anthrax
  clinical features of, 22–24
  diagnosis of, 24
  etiology of, 21–22
  investigations of, 25
  natural history of, 24
  treatment and follow-up of, 25
Apple jelly nodule, 41, 165
Ariboflavinosis, 226
Arsenical poisoning
  chronic, clinical features of, 239–240
  diagnosis of, 240–241
  etiology of, 238–239
  follow-up of, 242
  investigations of, 241
  treatment and follow-up of, 241–242
Avian tuberculosis, 36

Bacillus anthracis, 21, 22, 25
Bacillus anthrax, 21
Bacillus cereus, 25
Bacterial index (BI), 67–68
Bagdad boil, *see* Oriental sore
Bairnsdale bacillus, 78, 84
Bancroftian filariasis, 195
Beriberi, 224
Bilharzia, *see* Schistosomiasis

Biskra button, *see* Oriental sore
Bitot's spots, 222
Blastomyces dermatitidis, 141, 144
Blastomycosis, *see* North American
    blastomycosis and
    Paracoccidiomycosis
Borderline lepromatous (BL) disease,
    59–60
Borderline leprosy (BB), 49
  clinical features of, 58–60
  diagnosis of, 66
Borderline tuberculoid (BT) disease,
    58–59
Botryomycosis
  clinical features of, 130
  diagnosis of, 130–131
  etiology of, 129
  investigations of, 131
  treatment of, 131
Bovine tuberculosis, 36
Brazilian blastomycosis, *see*
    Paracoccidioidomycosis
Brazilian pemphigus foliaceous
  clinical features of, 233
  diagnosis of, 235–236
  etiology of, 232–233
  investigations of, 236
  natural history of, 234–235
  treatment of, 236–237
Brugia malayi, 195, 196
Brugia timori, 195
Buruli ulcer
  bacteriology of, 84
  clinical features of, 79, 81–83
  diagnosis of, 83–84
  etiology of, 78–79
  follow-up of, 87
  histology of, 84
  investigations of, 84
  local therapy for, 85
  natural history of, 83
  surgical treatment for, 85, 87
  systemic treatment for, 85

Camel's nose deformity, 170
Cellophane tape test, 243
Cellulitis, 201

Cephalosporium falciforme, 116
Cervical-facial infections, 125, *see also*
    Actinomycosis
Chiclero's ulcer, 176–177
Chloroquine
  for amebiasis, 181
  for lichen planus tropicus, 220
Chromomycosis
  clinical features of, 107
  diagnosis of, 108, 110
  etiology of, 106
  investigations of, 110–111
  natural history of, 107–108
  treatment of, 111
Cicatrical alopecia, 161
Cladosporium werneckii, 95, 96, 106
Clinical index, 6–17
Clofazimine
  for Buruli ulcer, 85
  for leprosy, 71
  for Lobo's disease, 155
Cloxacillin, for botryomycosis, 131
Coccidioides immitis, 144
Coccobacillus mycetoides, 90
Corynebacterium diphtheriae, 91
Corynebacterium mycetoides, 90
Corynebacterium pyogenes, 83, 91
Corynebacterium pyogenes ulcers, 91–92
Cotrimoxazole, for Madura foot, 117
Crab yaws, 30, *see also* Yaws
Cutaneous anthrax, 22–23, *see also*
    Anthrax
Cutaneous schistosomiasis, 207
Cutaneous tuberculosis, 36–37, *see also*
    Tuberculosis, of skin

Dapsone
  for leprosy, 64, 69
  for Madura foot, 117
Daughter yaws, 29, *see also* Yaws
Déjérine's disease, 65
Diarrhea, bloody, 179
Diascopy, 243–244
Dietary deficiencies, 221–227
Diethylcarbamazine
  for filariasis, 198
  for onchoceeiasis, 193

Dihydroemetine, 181
Diiodohydroxyquin, 181
Diiodohydroxyquinoline, 182
Diphtheritic ulcer, 91
Dirofilaria immitis, 198
Downgrading
  lepromatous disease and, 62, 66
Dracunculosis
  clinical features of, 201
  diagnosis of, 201–202
  etiology of, 200–201
  investigations of, 202–203
  natural history of, 201
  prevention of, 203–204
  treatment of, 203
Dracunculus medinensis, 200
Dutz technique, 244

Ectropion, 142
Entamoeba histolytica, 178
Eosinophic lung, tropical, in filariasis,
  197
Epistaxis, 134, 167
Erythema necrotisans, 74–75
Erythema nodosum leprosum (ENL),
  63–65
  histopathology of, 68–69
  lepromatous disease and, 66
  treatment of, 72
Erythromycin
  for actinomycosis, 128
  for botryomycosis, 131
  for yaws, 35
Ethambutol, 45
Ethylstilbamidine, for rhinosporidosis,
  136
Exophiala werneckii, 95
Eye changes, in onchocerciasis, 191–192

Favus
  clinical features of, 101
  diagnosis of, 103
  etiology of, 101
  investigations of, 103–104
  natural history of, 101, 103
  treatment of, 104

Filariasis
  clinical features of, 196
  diagnosis of, 198
  eosinophic lung in, 197
  etiology of, 195–196
  investigation of, 198
  natural history of, 196–197
  prevention of, 199
  skin tests for, 198
  treatment of, 198–199
Fogo selvagem, 232
Fonsecaea compacta, 106
Fonsecaea dermatiditis, 95
Fonsecaea pedrosi, 106
Fonsecaea verucose, 106
Frambesia, 29
Frisch's bacilli, 140

Gangrene, synergistic bacterial, 84
Gilchrist's disease, 141–145
Griseofulvin
  for favus, 104
  for tinea imbricata, 100
Guinea-worm disease, *see* Dracunculosis
Gumma, 30–32

Hair follicles, destruction of, 101,
  103
Hebra's nose deformity, 139
Hemorrhagic papule, 22–23
Histoplasma capsulatum, 144
Hyperkeratosis, 34
Hyperplasia, 137–138
Hypopigmentation, in leprosy, 54

Ichthyosis, 75–76
Immunity, and leprosy, 48–49
Insect bite, 160
Isonicotinic acid hydrazide, 45

Jamarsan R, 236
Jaundice, 179

Kala-azar, 173
Katayama disease, 207
Keloidal blastomycosis, *see* Lobo's
    disease
Keloids, 154
Keratosis pilaris, 229
Ketoconazole
    for chromomycosis, 111
    for favus, 104
    for Lobo's disease, 155
    for Madura foot, 117
    for mucocutaneous leishmaniasis, 173
    for North American blastomycosis,
        144
    for paracoccidioidmycosis, 150
    for sporotrichosis, 123
    for tinea imbricata, 100
Klebsiella rhinoscleromatis, 137, 140
Kwashiorkor, 221–222

Leishman-Donovan bodies, 159
Leishmania braziliensis, 170
Leishmania braziliensis guyanensis, 177
Leishmania donovani, 173
Leishmania major, 160
Leishmania mexicana, 176
Leishmania tropica, 160
Leishmaniasis, 159–177
Lepra bonita, 74
Lepra reactions, 61
Lupoid leishmaniasis, 167, *see also*
        Anergic leishmaniasis
Lepromatosis, diffuse, 74
Lepromatous leprosy (LL), 49
    clinical features of, 56–58
    diagnosis of, 66
Lepromin test, 69, 245
Leprosy, *see also Specific types*
    anergic patients and, 49
    bacteriology of, 67–68
    clinical features of, 51–52, 53–60
    diagnosis of, 65–66
    downgrading, 62
    etiology of, 48–49, 51
    follow-up of, 73
    histopathology of, 68–69

immunologic background and, 48
incomplete immunity and, 48–49
incubation period, 60–61
indeterminate, 73–74
investigations of, 67–69
natural history of, 60–65
reactions in, 61
reversal reactions in, 62
skin ulceration and, 75
spectrum of, 49, 51
sulfone-resistant, 69
treated, progress in, 62–63
treatment of, 69, 71–72
untreated, progress of, 61
variants of, 73–76
Leprosy alopecia, 75
Leprosy skin smear, 245–248
Lichen planus tropicus
    clinical features of, 216–217
    diagnosis of, 217–218
    etiology of, 215–216
    investigations of, 218
    treatment of, 218, 220
Lobo's disease
    clinical features of, 152–153
    diagnosis of, 153–154
    etiology of, 152
    investigations of, 154
    treatment of, 155
Loboa loboi, 152
Lucio phenomenon, 74–75
Lumpy jaw, 124
Lupoid leishmaniasis
    clinical features of, 165
    diagnosis of, 165–166
    investigations of, 166
    natural history of, 165
    treatment of, 166
Lupus vulgaris, 39, 41
    diagnosis of, 43
Lymphostasis verrucosa, 63, 108

Madarosis, 57–58, 167
Madura foot
    clinical features of, 113
    diagnosis of, 115–116

etiology of, 112–113
investigations of, 116
natural history of, 114–115
treatment of, 117
Madurella grisea, 116
Madurella mycetomi, 116
Mal morado, 189
Malayan filariasis, 195
Malignancy, arsenic ingestion and, 239
Malignant pustule, 22
Marasmus, 224
Matchstick test, 244
Mazzotti test, 193
Mebendazole, 198
Meleney's burrowing ulcer, 84
Metrifonate, 210
Metronidazole
   for amebiasis, 182
   for dracunculosis, 201
   for tropical ulcers, 90
Micrococcus mycetoides, 90
Mikulicz' cells, 140
Miliary tuberculosis, 38–39
Montenegro test, 164
Morphologic index (MI), 64
   definition of, 68
   drug therapy and, 69, 71
   useful techniques, 24
Mossy foot, 63, 108, 196
Mother yaw, 29, *see also* Yaws
Mucocutaneous leishmaniasis
   clinical features of, 170–171
   diagnosis of, 172
   investigations of, 172
   natural history of, 171–172
   treatment of, 172–173
Mulberry erosions, 146, 148
Mycetoid desert sore, 90
Mycetomas, deep, 114, *see also* Madura
   foot
Mycobacterium balnei, 43, 44
Mycobacterium leprae, 44, 48
   bacteriology of 66–67
   ENL and, 72
   predilection for nervous tissue, 51
   signs and symptoms from, 65–66
Mycobacterium tuberculosis, 36, 44

Mycobacterium ulcerans, 44
   bacteriology of, 84
   phenomena unique to, 79

Neural leprosy, 49
   clinical features of, 51–52, 54
   diagnosis of, 65
Night blindness, 228
Nikolsky's sign, 248
N-methylglucamine antimoniae, 172
Nocardia asteroides, 124
Nocardia brasiliensis, 124
Nocardia braziliensis, 116
North American blastomycosis
   clinical features of, 142
   diagnosis of, 143
   etiology of, 141
   investigations of, 144
   natural history of, 142–143
   treatment of, 144–145

Onchocerca volvulus, 188
Onchocerciasis
   clinical features of, 188–192
   diagnosis of, 192–193
   etiology of, 188
   investigations of, 193
   natural history of, 192
   prevention of, 194
   treatment of, 193–194
Onchocerciasis skin snip, 248
Oriental sore
   clinical features of, 160–161
   diagnosis of, 163
   etiology of, 160
   investigations of, 163–164
   natural history of, 161, 163
   treatment of, 164–165
Orthopedic surgery, for leprosy, 72
Oxamniquine, 210

Paracoccidioides braziliensis, 146, 149–
   150

Paracoccidioidomycosis
  clinical features of, 146, 148
  diagnosis of, 149
  etiology of, 146
  investigations of, 149–150
  natural history of, 148
  treatment and follow-up of, 150
Parrot's beak deformity, 171
Pellagra, 224–226
Pellagra necklace, 225
Pemphigus foliaceous, 232, *see also*
      Brazilian pemphigus
      foliaceous
Penicillin
  for actinomycosis, 128
  for yaws, 34–35
Phialophora jeanselmei, 116
Phrynoderma
  clinical features of, 229
  diagnosis of, 229, 231
  etiology of, 228
  treatment of, 231
Pian bois, 177
Plastic surgery, for leprosy, 72
Post-kala-azar dermal leishmaniasis
  clinical features of, 173
  diagnosis of, 176
  investigations of, 176
  natural history of, 173, 176
  treatment of, 176
Praziquantel, 210
Prednisone
  for Brazilian pemphigus foliaceous,
      236
  for erythema· nodosum leprosum,
      72
  for leprosy, 71–72
Promastigote, 159
Pseudomonas aeruginosa, 129
Pullularia werneckii, 106
Pulmonary anthrax, 24, *see also*
      Anthrax
Pulmonary blastomycosis, 142–143
Pyrimethamine, 186

Quinacrine, 236

Raspberry papule, 29
Reversal reaction
  lepromatous disease and, 66
  leprosy and, 62
Rhinoscleroma
  clinical features of, 137–138
  diagnosis of, 139–140
  etiology of, 137
  investigations of, 140
  natural history of, 138–139
  treatment of, 140
Rhinosporidiosis
  clinical features of, 134
  diagnosis of, 134–135
  etiology of, 133
  investigations of, 135
  natural history of, 134
  treatment of, 136
Rhinosporidium seeberi, 133
Ridley-Jopling classification, of leprosy,
      49, 51
Rifampin
  for Buruli ulcer, 85
  for leprosy, 71
  for tuberculosis, 45
River blindness, 187

Salak, 161
Sandfly bite, 160
Schistosoma haematobium, 205, 206
Schistosoma japonicum, 205, 206
Schistosoma mansoni, 205, 206
Schistosome dermatitis, 207
Schistosomiasis
  clinical features of, 206–207
  cutaneous, 207
  diagnosis of, 209–210
  etiology of, 206
  invasive, 206–207
  investigations of, 210
  natural history of, 207–209
  prevention of, 211
  treatment of, 210
  urticarial, 207
Schistosoma ova, viability test of, 248–
      249

Scrofuloderma, 38
Scurvy, 227
Simulium damnosum, 187
Simulium ochraceum, 189
Sodium stibogluconate, for Oriental
    sore, 164
South American blastomycosis, *see*
    paracoccidioidomycosis
Spiramycin, for toxoplasmosis, 186
Splendore-Hoeppli phenomenon, 122
Sporothrix schenckii, 118
Sporotrichosis
    clinical features of, 119
    diagnosis of, 122
    etiology of, 118
    investigations of, 122
    natural history of, 119, 122
    treatment of, 123
Scrofuloderma, diagnosis of, 43
Staphylococcus aureus, 129
Staphylococcus pyogenes, 129
Steroid therapy, for lichen planus
    tropicus, 220
Stibophen, 176
Strawberry polyp, 134–135
Streptomyces madurae, 116
Streptomyces somaliensis, 116
Streptomycin, 140
Sulfadiazine, 186
Sulfone therapy, for leprosy, 64
    resistence of, 69
Suramin
    for filariasis, 198
    for onchoceeiasis, 194
Synergistic bacterial gangrene, 84

Tetracycline
    for actinomycosis, 128
    for anthrax, 25
    for botryomycosis, 131
    for yaws, 35
Thalidomide, 72
Thiabendazole, 201
Thiamin, 224
Thoracic actinomycosis, 125–126, *see*
    also Actinomycosis

Tinea captitis, 100
Tinea favosa, *see* Favus
Tinea imbricata
    clinical features of, 97
    diagnosis of, 100
    etiology of, 97
    natural history of, 99
    treatment of, 100
Tinea nigra
    clinical features of, 96
    diagnosis of, 96
    etiology of, 95
    treatment of, 96–97
Tineas tropical, 97–104
Tokelau ringworm, *see* Tinea imbricata
Toxoplasma gondii, 183
Toxoplasmosis
    clinical features of, 184
    diagnosis of, 185
    etiology of, 183
    investigations of, 185–186
    natural history of, 184–185
    treatment of, 186
Treponema carateum, 27, 34
Treponema pallidum, 27, 34
Treponema pertenue, 27, 28, 34
Treponema vincenti, 89
Tretinoin, 231
Trichophyton concentricum, 97, 99
Trichophyton schoenleinii, 100, 101,
    103
Tropical ulcers, 88–92
    treatment of, 90
Tropicaloid ulcer, 90–91
Tuberculoid leprosy (TT), 49
    clinical features of, 54
    diagnosis of, 55, 65–66
    histopathology of, 68
Tuberculosis, of skin
    bacteriology of, 44
    clinical features of, 37–39, 41, 43
    diagnosis of, 43
    etiology of, 36–37
    investigations of, 44–45
    natural history of, 43
    pathology of, 44
    treatment and follow-up of, 45–46

Tuberculosis verrucosa cutis, diagnosis
    of, 38, 43
Tuberculous chancre, 37–38
Tuberculous lesions, 41, 43
Tuberculous ulcers, 38
Tzanck test, 249

Ulcer
    Buruli, *see* Buruli ulcer
    buttock, 83
    Corynebacterium pyogenes, 91–92
    diphtheritic, 91
    Meleney's burrowing, 84
    serpiginous, 31–32
    tropical, 88–92
    tropicaloid, 90–91
    tuberculous, 38
Urticarial schistosomiasis, 207

Veldt sore, 91
Vincent's organisms, 89
Vitamin A deficiency, 224
    phrynoderma and, 228

Vitamin B deficiencies, 224–226
    treatment of, 226
Vitamin C deficiency, 227

Whitfield's lotion
    for tinea imbricata, 100
    for tinea nigra, 96
Wood's light, 249
Wuchereria bancrofti, 195, 196
Wuchereria pacifica, 195

Yaws
    clinical features of, 28–32
    crab, 30
    daughter, 29
    diagnosis of, 33–34
    early, 29–30
    etiology of, 27–28
    investigation of, 34
    late, 30–32
    mother, 29
    natural history of, 32–33
    treatment of, 34–35